D0979150

THRIVE

THRIVE

How Better Mental Health Care
Transforms Lives and Saves Money

Richard Layard
and David M. Clark

WITHDRAWN

Princeton University Press   *Princeton & Oxford*

Copyright © 2014 by Richard Layard and David M. Clark
Original edition first published in the United Kingdom as
Thrive: The Power of Evidence-Based Psychological Therapies
by Penguin Books Ltd, London
Requests for permission to reproduce material from this work
should be sent to Permissions, Princeton University Press
Published in the United States by Princeton University Press,
41 William Street, Princeton, New Jersey 08540

press.princeton.edu

All Rights Reserved

ISBN 978-0-691-16963-7
Library of Congress Control Number: 2015936812

British Library Cataloging-in-Publication Data is available

This book has been composed in Sabon Next, Scala Sans,
and Baucher

Printed on acid-free paper. ∞

Printed in the United States of America

1 3 5 7 9 10 8 6 4 2

TO MOLLY AND ANKE

CONTENTS

Contents

FOREWORD

This book is an inspiring success story and a stirring call to further action. Its message is as compelling as it is important: the social costs of mental illness are terribly high, and the costs of effective treatments are surprisingly low.

Some time ago, my colleagues and I set out to measure how much suffering there is in our society. We conducted several studies in which a large number of people provided a description of their day; they broke their working hours into episodes, for each of which they specified the starting time and ending time. For each episode they indicated the main activity in which they had been engaged at that time, and they rated the extent to which they had experienced various emotions. We classified as "suffering" any episode in which at least one of the negative emotions (for example, "depressed," "worried," or "angry") was rated as more intense than all the positive emotions in the list (for example, "happy," "enjoying myself"). We then computed for each individual the total duration of bad episodes and the fraction of the day in which she had suffered. We collected responses from many hundreds of women in several countries (United States, France, and Denmark) and observed that the average time spent suffering was between 15% and 20% of the waking day. We also found that the distribution of suffering among individuals was grossly unequal. About half the respondents indicated no suffering at all. But the 10% who reported the most pain accounted for nearly half the total suffering that we recorded in our sample.

The conclusion was stark: A significant minority of the population is in almost constant psychological pain. A more positive conclusion was that if we wish to reduce suffering in our society, we should concentrate on alleviating the emotional (and physical) pain of the most afflicted individuals. The sufferers at any one time include people who have suffered a calamity of some kind—a painful divorce, the death of a relative. There is not much that society can do about that. But the sufferers also include a substantial number of people who are chronically in a bad emotional state, without an obvious trigger for their grief. These are the mentally ill, and mental illness is treatable.

My colleagues and I, all American academics, noted the fact that these observations could be used to support a policy of intervening to mitigate the effects of the scourge of mental illness. But we did not know how to go about it, and we did nothing but talk. The authors of this book live in another society, they are made of different cloth, and they combined their exceptional skills and connection to tackle the problem head on. Richard Layard is an economist (as well as a Member of the House of Lords) and David Clark is a professor of psychology at Oxford University. They were well aware of the prevalence of psychological illness in the United Kingdom and of the enormous toll that psychological disorders inflict, on the afflicted individuals, on their families, and on society as a whole through lost productivity and higher welfare costs.

David Clark and Richard Layard also knew that something could be done about mental illness. Clark is an expert in the one form of psychological intervention whose distinctive benefits have been established by systematic objective research. This is *cognitive behavior therapy*, a relatively brief course of focused conversations between a patient and a professional, in which patients learn new ways of thinking about their problems and new approaches to controlling their emotions. Cognitive behavior therapy is not a panacea. It works much better in some problems than others: it is, for example, very effective at alleviating anxiety and eating disorders and in combating depression, but is less likely to bring relief for psychotic conditions. Where it is effective, however, cognitive behavior therapy can be helpful indeed. Complete or partial recovery from incapacitating symptoms can be achieved with many patients—more than half in good clinics—in a few meetings conducted once or twice a week. The benefits to the individuals and their families are obvious. The benefit to society is also impressive: recovered patients return to work, contribute to the economy and pay taxes, and they cease to be a burden on other taxpayers.

Combining the power of their skills and positions, Richard Layard and David Clark caused a significant change in the health policies in the United Kingdom, securing substantial government support for the training of many thousands of professionals in the science and practice of a range of evidence-based psychological therapies. They also ensured expanded financial support of the National Health Service for the treatment of mental illness. Very importantly, the system they created involved careful monitoring of the outcomes of treatment. Interventions with patients are graded on a scale of success from complete recovery to total failure, and statistics are kept that enable the system to track the quality of care in different centers and the efficacy of treatments for different forms of mental illness. The statistics, in turn, inform future policies and practices. It is already clear that the increased availability of evidence-based psychological therapies in the United Kingdom is a major success, in which human suffering is reduced at no cost to taxpayers—because direct expenditures are fully compensated by the accelerated return of patients to an active role in the economy.

The unprecedented success story that Richard Layard and David Clark document in this book has implications for any society in which mental illness is a serious problem—and that means every society. The demonstrated effectiveness of modern psychological therapies is relevant to individual sufferers and their families in the United States, where these treatments are well known. The message of this book is also relevant to policy makers and government officials at all levels, city, state and federal: the availability of evidence-based psychological therapies should be increased and supported by public funds, on the expectation that the overall financial benefits of the program will be positive. The exact details of implementation will vary from place to place, but the principle is clear: something can be done to reduce human suffering, with large social benefits and no social costs. As was the case in the United Kingdom, the policy message of the book should attract support from everyone, regardless of politics. The potential for broad agreement on a public intervention of proven efficacy and cost-effectiveness is a welcome change in a polarized society. As this book illustrates, ideology is not the only way to define policies that people can be enthusiastic about. Carefully documented facts can sometimes tell an inspiring story that everyone should hear.

DANIEL KAHNEMAN
Professor Emeritus, Princeton University

PREFACE

One of us is an economist and the other a clinical psychologist. We met ten years ago and at once began discussing one of the great injustices of our time. If people are physically ill they generally get treated, but if they are mentally ill they usually do not. Yet really good treatments exist.

So together we lobbied the British government until it launched its landmark program, Improving Access to Psychological Therapies. Since it began, we have both been advisers to the program. It still has a long way to go, but it has already changed the lives of hundreds of thousands of people. According to the journal *Nature* it is "world-beating,"[1] and countries around the world are already looking to it for guidance.

This book draws on our experience—of making the case for mental health and of constructive policy development. It is also the indirect product of a whole community of people who have been struggling to bring evidence-based psychological therapy to the millions of people who need it.

Our book sets out the nature and scale of the problem, the case for action, and the outline of a solution. People with mental health problems should have the same access to treatment as people who are physically ill. It is morally right that they should, and it is also vital for our economy and for the functioning of our society.

In the last fifty years there has been massive social progress on many fronts. Yet much misery remains, because we have failed to address the inner psychological sources of distress. That is now a central challenge for the twenty-first century.

RICHARD LAYARD AND DAVID CLARK,
February 2015

PART ONE

The Problem

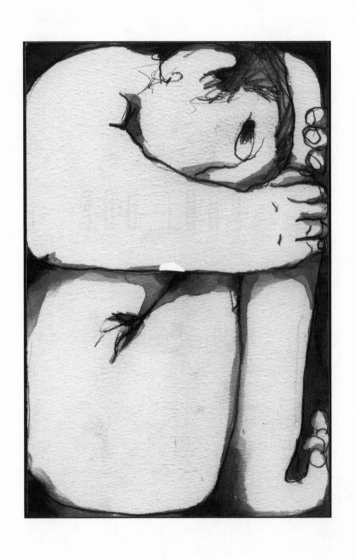

1 * What's the Problem?

I was much too far out all my life
And not waving but drowning

Stevie Smith, "Not Waving but Drowning"

Dennis Stevenson is a well-known businessman, and has occasional bouts of depression. This is how he describes them. "I once broke my leg in ten places. As I was taken to hospital, someone shut the door on my leg. You can imagine the pain. But I can tell you the pain of depression is many times worse: it is excruciating."

Mental pain is as real as physical pain. It is experienced in the same areas of the brain as physical pain and is often more disabling. Yet these two types of pain are not treated equally. While nearly everyone who is physically ill gets treatment, two in three of those who are mentally ill do not. If your bone is broken you are treated automatically, but if your spirit is broken you are not.

This is a shocking form of discrimination, which occurs in every health care system in the world. It is particularly shocking because we have very good treatments for the most common mental health problems, which are depression and crippling anxiety disorders. The treatments—modern psychological therapy and drugs when appropriate—are not expensive. And the economics are striking.

Treating mental health problems produces extraordinary savings—fewer people on welfare benefits, and fewer people being treated for physical illnesses made worse by mental illness. So on any reasonable estimates the treatments pay for themselves. They cost society nothing. And yet they are provided to under a third of those who need them. That is a great injustice and a gross inefficiency. And it is the main reason we have written this book—the pain of untreated mental health problems, and the fact that they can be treated at little or no cost.

There is also a wider issue. The last fifty years have seen enormous progress in advanced societies—less absolute poverty, better physical health, more education, and better housing. And yet in the United States, Britain, and many other countries, there is almost as much misery as there was fifty years ago[1]—at least as many social problems and more family conflict, more crime, and more antisocial behavior. Dealing with the externals of income, education, physical illness, and housing has not been enough to produce happier or more orderly lives. We have left something out—the inner person. Mental health is something that requires deliberate cultivation and expert help when it goes wrong. If our society had better mental health, we should all gain. That is the second reason we have written this book: the huge social cost of mental illness.

The facts we lay out are in many cases quite remarkable—indeed, after many years in the field some of them still amaze even us. Here are the main questions we investigate.[2]

How Many Suffer?

Mental illness is the great hidden problem in our societies, so most people are amazed when they hear the scale of it.[3] In the Western world today one in six of all adults suffers from depression or a crippling anxiety disorder. Roughly a third of households currently include someone who is mentally ill.

When people ask us what we work on and we say mental health, the reply is almost always, "Oh, my son . . . ," or "my mother . . . ," or sometimes, "I have to admit that I . . . ," but then usually, "and please don't tell anyone." (This is particularly true when it's a politician.) In America, more people commit suicide than are killed in road accidents.[4]

Mental illness is not only common, but it can also be truly disabling through its impact on people's ability to care for themselves, to function socially, to get around, and to avoid physical and mental pain. In that sense, depression is on average 50% more disabling than angina, asthma, arthritis, or diabetes.

So here is an extraordinary fact. When in 2008 the World Health Organization measured the scale of illness and allowed for its severity, they found that in rich countries mental illness accounted for nearly 40% of all illness.[5] By contrast, stroke, cancer, heart disease, lung disease, and diabetes accounted for less than 20%. Figure 1.1 says it all.

Mental illness is extremely difficult to adapt to—much more so than most physical illness except for unremitting pain.[6] It is terrible for those who experience it. But it is also bad for business, since it gives rise to nearly half of all days off sick. And it is bad for taxpayers, since mental illness accounts for nearly half of all the people who live on disability benefits. And it is bad for insurers since mental health problems add 50% to a person's bill for physical health care.

Given all this, you would think that mental illness would be high on the priorities of every insurer and every government's department of health. But not so. In 2007 we met

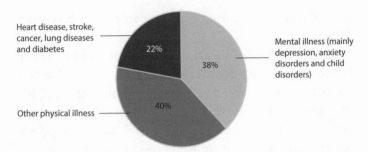

Figure 1.1. Mental illness is 38% of all ill health in rich countries.

with Britain's new secretary of state for health after he had been in his job for three weeks. At the end of our meeting he said, "Something has struck me. I've been in post for three weeks and gone to about forty meetings, but I have not so far heard the phrase 'mental health.'"

The situation is similar with employers. In January 2012 the World Economic Forum was having its usual snow-bound conference in Davos. This included a meeting of the Workplace Wellness Alliance—a group of sixty of the world's most enlightened employers. The meeting was about the health challenges facing employers, and there were detailed presentations on cardiovascular disease, diabetes, lung problems, cancer, and musculoskeletal issues—but there was nothing on mental illness, even though it causes so much sickness absence. People just don't want to talk about it.

Do They Get Help?

Given this, it is not surprising that most mental illness goes untreated.[7] While most people with physical illness are in treatment, this is true for fewer than one in three people with mental illness. This figure applies throughout the advanced world, and even for major depressions the figure is under a half in the United States, Britain, and continental Europe. If your pancreas is not working you automatically get treatment, but if your mind has been disordered for decades you do not.

What could account for this shocking failure? Stigma is one reason. People are ashamed of being mentally ill. They feel that, while physical illness is an act of the gods, mental illness is in some way their own fault. Relatives are also full of guilt. In most countries no effective lobby exists on behalf of people with mental illness, as it does for heart disease, cancer, and the like.

But another important reason is simply technological lag. Many people don't know that we have new treatments for mental illness that are just as effective as the treatments for many physical illnesses.

Can They Be Treated Effectively?

This is a new situation.[8] Until the 1950s there were no scientifically validated treatments for mental illness. But in that decade there were major discoveries of drugs that could help to control psychotic symptoms (the antipsychotics) and depression (the antidepressants). Even so, many sufferers are averse to drugs, often because of their side effects, and that partly explains the low numbers in treatment. But then in the 1960s and 1970s came major breakthroughs in psychological therapy. The most important of these was what is now called cognitive behavioral therapy (CBT), which relies on the fact that thoughts affect feelings, and that good mental habits can be systematically built up step by step. CBT is certainly not the only therapy that works, and it does not always work. But it has been evaluated so much more often than any other therapy that we can speak with certainty about its average overall effects. These have now been established in hundreds of randomized clinical trials of exactly the same kind as those used in testing any medical treatment.

The general finding is that around 50% of people treated with CBT for depression or anxiety conditions recover during treatment, and many others improve significantly. For depression, CBT is as effective as drugs in the short run, and more effective in preventing the recurrence of depression down the road. For anxiety, CBT is even more impressive. Many people with conditions like social phobia, panic disorder, or obsessive-compulsive disorder have had their condition for decades, but if successfully treated they are mostly cured for life.

A leading hero of this "psychological revolution" is the psychiatrist Aaron Beck of the University of Pennsylvania. He began as a psychoanalyst and wanted to make psychoanalysis scientific. So he designed a study to confirm one of its central tenets—that depression is due to unconscious hostility that has been repressed and directed against yourself.[9] With a team of colleagues, he compared the dreams of depressed and nondepressed patients. Contrary to his expectations, it turned out that the depressed patients had less hostility in their dreams than the other patients did. However, their dreams did seem to be quite similar to how they were actually thinking when awake. They saw themselves as victims; people or circumstances were against them; they felt thwarted, rejected, or deserted.

Beck focused all his efforts on what his patients were actually thinking—getting them to observe the automatic thoughts that were part of their thinking style.[10] He sat facing them to try and detect their unspoken thoughts. When a cloud passed over a face, he would say, "What was going through your mind just then?" It turned out that the thinking style of depressed people included catastrophizing (thinking the worst), black-and-white judgments, and overgeneralizing from a single bad experience. To help his patients, Beck trained them to examine their thoughts and how they might be biased or distorted. To his surprise, they often stopped coming to see him within twelve sessions, saying they had had all they needed.

Another hero of the "psychological revolution" was Joseph Wolpe, a South African doctor who moved to Philadelphia. He also trained in psychoanalysis but was frustrated at the slow pace of treatment. He read the work of the Russian physiologist Ivan Pavlov, which showed that fears in animals could be extinguished by exposing the animal to the object of its fears in a gradual way. Wolpe applied this form of behavior therapy to his clients and, like Beck, found they recovered quickly. Beck and Wolpe had essential insights that became combined in the development of cognitive behavioral therapies. To ensure that their new treatments could have reliable results, they developed manuals of good practice that any well-trained practitioner with enough empathy could apply. And to measure effectiveness they developed rigorous scales of measurement and used these in scientific randomized trials to find out what proportion of patients recovered. The resulting recovery rates of 50% or more now offer hope to millions of people worldwide.

There are certainly other therapies that can also be extremely effective. They need to be systematically developed and tested. So when the history is written we shall hopefully see how CBT paved the way for other, perhaps more powerful, therapies. But for the moment, what CBT has done is to bring psychological therapy to a point where it can claim scientifically to be able to transform lives. It will be seen to have changed our culture forever.

One striking fact about modern treatments (be they drugs or therapy) is the rigor with which outcomes are measured. This is far from the vague, less structured and more prolonged therapy that many doctors tend to despise. It is science of a high order, based on randomized controlled trials and capable of replication, with success rates as high as in the majority of treatments available for physical illnesses. But not enough people know this, and evidence-based psychological therapy is hard to access in almost every country.

Are the Treatments Costly?

This is not because the treatments are costly.[11] A standard course of cognitive behavioral therapy involves up to sixteen one-hour sessions, one-on-one—with the average number of sessions nearer to ten. The total cost is about $2,000. With a 50% success rate for a serious condition, this is good value for money. And that is why it is recommended for almost all mental health conditions in the official guidelines for the British National Health Service.[12]

But actually the economics is even better than that. There are some striking lessons here for those who finance the health care system. It turns out that mental health has a huge effect on physical health, and thus on health care costs. The effects on life expectancy are extraordinary: depression reduces your length of life as much as smoking does (and not mainly through suicide). And while you're alive, depression and anxiety conditions increase your visits to the family doctor and to specialists. Conversely, controlled trials show that if you get psychological therapy, you go to the doctor for physical ailments much less often than those who remain untreated. The resulting savings are large enough to fully cover the cost of the psychological therapy. For the health care authorities and insurers, this is a win-win situation: pay for more psychological therapy and it will cost you nothing because of the savings on physical health care. The finances of health care actually improve through spending more on therapy.

So too do the finances of the welfare system, because many people with mental illness cannot work. When psychological therapy becomes more widely available, some of those who use it will be people who are on welfare or in danger of losing their job. As a result of the therapy, more of them will be at work and fewer on welfare benefits. Robust calculations show that the resulting savings on benefits and lost taxes will exceed the cost of the psychological therapy. There is a double payoff—the cost of the therapy is repaid twice over, both in savings on physical health care and in savings on benefits and lost taxes.

Despite all this, those who finance health care are generally resistant to providing the extra resources needed. That is the main reason why so few people are in treatment: it is the funders above all who are to blame.

Early Intervention?

The case for more help becomes even stronger when we shift from adults to children.[13] Here again good treatments exist, but they are not widely available in most countries. The scale of undertreatment is as bad for youngsters as it is for adults: only one in four young people with mental health problems is in treatment.

The myopia here is quite extraordinary, since half of all mental illness in adult life began in childhood. Moreover, child mental illness is a cause of so many of our social problems. Mentally ill children are much more likely than others to avoid school, to take drugs, and to self-harm. And when they become adults (if they had "conduct disorder" in youth) they are much more likely to be arrested for a crime, to become teenage parents, to get divorced, and to live off benefits. This brings us to our second, wider theme—the impact of mental illness on society at large.

A Better Society?

In the darkest days of World War II, Winston Churchill commissioned Sir William Beveridge to review the future of social policy in Britain. In his famous report, which determined postwar policy, Beveridge identified five giants that were responsible for the ills of society. They were Want, Idleness, Ignorance, Squalor, and Disease, or in modern parlance: poverty, unemployment, undereducation, poor housing, and physical illness. Since then we have made huge progress against all five of these giants, except at times unemployment. Yet our society is no happier now than it was then. We have more broken families, more disturbed children, and more crime.[14] One major reason is that the human factor inside each of us has remained much the same. We have tackled the external problems but not the one inside, the sixth giant: the evil of mental illness.

That is where we have gone wrong. We have assumed that most problems are external. Many of them of course are, but not all. Problems of depression, anxiety, and dysfunctional personality are as old as the human race. What is new is that in the last fifty years we have developed major ways of addressing these problems.

We have therapies that people want and that are not expensive. And they have good success rates as measured by rigorous clinical trials. But they are simply not available to most people. Our claim is that, if they were, we could have a truly better society.

This is not the only thing that needs doing—we also recommend preventive policies and major social changes.[15] But in the meantime there are millions suffering. We know how they could be helped, and what the results would be. Getting them the treatment they need is the top priority and the way we can be most sure of making a real difference. That is the main claim we want to establish in this book.

To do so, we ask a series of questions, chapter by chapter. In part one we look at how mental illness affects people's lives, and the lives of those around them. We also ask what causes it. Then in part two we turn to what can be done about it. Excellent treatments exist, and these now need to be provided on a massive scale. England's Improving Access to Psychological Therapies program is one example of what can be done.[16] And there is also a whole raft of changes that can reduce the chances of mental illness in the first place.

The time is ripe for a radical rethink. Mental illness blights so many lives and causes so many problems. But there is great good news: it can be tackled, and it will not cost us an arm and a leg. Dealing with it, as one journalist has put it, is "a no-brainer."[17]

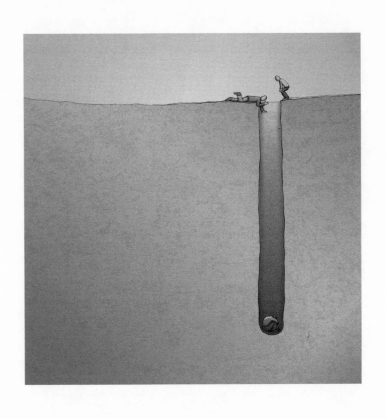

2 * What Is Mental Illness?

Depression is the most unpleasant thing I have ever
experienced.... It is that absence of being able to
envisage that you will ever be cheerful again. The absence
of hope.

J. K. Rowling

Gareth is a nice-looking man in his thirties with considerable personal charm. But for most of his twenties he was
totally housebound. He could not bear to be with other
people and thought he was so ugly that everyone would
laugh at him if they saw him. If he did go out, he had panic
attacks and would have to escape and hide away.

Such irrational fear and self-hatred is astonishing but not
uncommon. As a boy, Gareth, though a good student, had
been nervous in company, and he once wrote a school essay
about depression and thinking of killing himself. But it was
not till he started work that things became too much and
he found himself unable to cope. For the next seven years
he had no job. Through his family doctor he got eighteen
months of "psychodynamic" psychotherapy, in which he
reexplored his past life and his dysfunctional family—his
parents had split up when he was thirteen and he first lived
with his father, who could be quite violent, and then his
mother. But the therapist would not address his current
problems: the self-disgust and the social anxiety. He got no
better. Over the next two years he was referred to two more
psychologists, one of whose approach was again "person-
centered." But he found this treatment equally unhelpful.
Nor did any medication seem to help.

But then he saw a TV documentary called *Too Ugly for Love*. It was about "body dysmorphic disorder," the condition where you are convinced you are ugly and people will laugh at you. It felt exactly like how he felt. He sought out the therapist who presented the program and at last got himself diagnosed. After another three years of struggle, he was admitted to the therapist's residential clinic for anxiety disorders, for twelve weeks of CBT.

As Gareth put it, "within eight weeks my life had changed." Later he wrote,

> I am enjoying for the first time in my life things that most people take for granted, such as walking in a crowd of people and feeling relaxed and part of society, speaking aloud in a classroom setting, or sitting in a café enjoying a snack. It often feels as though I have been reborn, the world now transformed from a place filled with fear and threat to one full of possibility and excitement.[1]

He immediately began voluntary work, and then trained as a therapist. He now practices full time. If you met him, you would not believe the ordeal he has been through, except that at times it makes him cry to talk about it.

Lisa is fifty-three. Her anxieties began early, soon after her three-year-old sister died of cancer. She worried about one thing after another, and by the age of fourteen she had checking rituals to control her worries. By the time she got her art degree, her mind was obsessed with the idea that she was going to kill someone. She wanted to see inside their brains, and to do this she would have to kill. To deal with these obsessive thoughts, she went into a clinic, but they only dealt with how her thoughts might reflect the death of her little sister and other childhood events. She acquired no way of managing her thoughts. For years she was unable to work. She became an alcoholic and walked out on her baby son. Medication did not help. But eventually, at fifty, she went into a clinic specializing in the treatment of obsessive-compulsive disorder (OCD).

Three years later, this is what she writes:

> With the techniques I learnt at the specialist OCD unit I feel capable of dealing with the ruminations that do pop up, and no longer feel a need to consult psychotherapists. I've completely left behind any desire to return to alcohol.
>
> I am a non-perfect roly-poly middle-aged woman of fifty-three but I now feel like I'm an emotional millionaire! Before this I felt I was at core a bad egg; I left the specialist OCD unit as an all-right egg, with ambitions for the future—more of a free-range egg, more mentally flexible. My son wrote recently on his birthday card to me, "Not even a dinosaur could take me away from you!"[2]

On February 28, 2006, Captain Kevin Ivison was leading his bomb disposal team along a high road in Iraq. A massive bomb exploded, killing two of his friends in front of his eyes. A violent crowd of Iraqis assembled behind his remaining vehicles, blocking retreat. But in front he could see another massive bomb. If he attempted to dismantle it, it could be exploded by remote radio control or he could be killed by sniper fire. Terror gripped him. He was sure he was going to die. Even so he went forward to immobilize the bomb. It took twenty minutes, but he succeeded and escaped with the rest of his team. However, his nerves were shattered, and he left the army. Although he was awarded a medal for bravery, he still felt that his friends' deaths were his fault. While awake, he could think about nothing else except that day, and asleep he had the most violent night-mares. All he could think about was death and the fear of death. Formerly the best of company, he had become sullen and intolerant of everything, from people to noise.

He knew he needed treatment, but it was not until four years later that he found it. He had twelve long sessions of CBT in which he remembered every moment of that day in a totally safe environment, with no judgments made of any sort. And through therapy, he came to tolerate the ir-ritations of daily life. As he put it, "within two months of starting I felt like a completely different person and by the end I was—almost—the 'old' me again."[3]

Anxiety

Gareth, Lisa, and Kevin are typical of millions of people—men and women—across the world suffering from anxiety disorders of various kinds. When humans evolved in the sa-vannah alongside other dangerous animals, those humans who were more jumpy were more likely to survive. Anxiety was functional. But in modern conditions, excessive worry becomes dysfunctional. Most of us worry more than is good for us, but there is a whole spectrum of worrying and obses-sion. In roughly 8% of people the degree of anxiety is crippling enough to need professional help.[4] Such people are suffering from "anxiety disorders."

In some people the anxiety is quite *generalized*. They worry about many things; find it difficult to concentrate, to sit still, or to sleep properly. This can produce fatigue and extreme distress. But specific anxieties are often more crippling. The most common of these are panic attacks, social phobia, obsessive-compulsive disorder, and posttraumatic stress disorder.

People having *panic attacks* believe they are going to die, or faint, or have a heart attack, or a stroke, or go mad. They experience some bodily sensation that they believe is a signal of danger. This sets off their "fight or flight" mechanism and their heart races. They never do die, but the fear is so intense that even the fear of an attack can induce an attack. People with such fears are often unable to leave the house for fear of what might happen—they become agoraphobic. One-fifth of people who have panic disorder attempt to kill themselves.[5]

People with *social phobia* believe other people will think them boring or inept. They constantly monitor the impression they are making on people, and this self-consciousness makes things even worse. They often blush, sweat, or shake. When things get bad enough they just hide, as Gareth did for all those years.

People with *obsessive-compulsive disorder* have very specific thoughts or behaviors they cannot prevent, even though they want to. Lisa is an example of someone with obsessive thoughts. The most common thoughts are of killing someone or committing some other dreadful deed. Compulsive behaviors include repeated washing of hands or repeated checking of whether doors are locked—often for more than an hour on end. These kinds of thoughts and behaviors can become completely disabling.

And, finally, *posttraumatic stress disorder* can affect anyone, like Kevin, who has had a specific shock that constantly recurs in his/her thoughts or that some experience or other brings back. Such people typically become highly sensitive, jumpy, and irritable, in a way that can cripple relationships at home and at work.

Anxiety conditions, especially social phobia, often start in childhood. Once they begin, most anxiety conditions tend to persist over long periods of time. In one survey of patients the average person had had their condition for more than seventeen years.[6] But equally, once the anxiety is successfully treated, recovery tends to persist.[7]

Depression

Depression is more episodic, but equally devastating. Lewis Wolpert is a distinguished academic, whom all that know him experience as extremely positive. Yet at the age of sixty-five he was struck down by a major depression. As he says,

> It was the worst experience of my life. More terrible even than watching my wife die of cancer. I am ashamed to admit that my depression felt worse than her death, but it is true. I was in a state that bears no resemblance to anything I had experienced before. It was not just feeling low, depressed in the commonly used sense of the word. I was seriously ill. I was totally self-involved, negative, and thought about suicide most of the time. I could not think properly, let alone work,

and wanted to remain curled up in bed all day. I could not ride my bicycle or go out on my own. I had panic attacks if left alone. And there were numerous physical symptoms—my whole skin would seem to be on fire and I developed uncontrollable twitches. Every new physical sign caused extreme anxiety. I was terrified, for example, that I would be unable to urinate. Sleep was impossible without sleeping pills: these only worked for a few hours, and when I woke up I felt worse. The future was hopeless. I was convinced that I would never work again or recover. There was the strong fear that I might go mad. And suicide was the solution.

Lewis believes that his depression originated from the physical effect of changing the drug that was prescribed for his heart arrhythmia, together with fear of retirement. But then the feelings took over. He began drug treatment but was overwhelmed with the desire to kill himself. The only solution was the safety of a hospital, but for weeks the agony continued. Then he improved enough to go home, but he could still not bear to be left alone. So he embarked on a course of CBT. He had been offered CBT in his blackest hour and it hadn't helped. But now he found it "tremendously helpful." Eventually he became able to work and resume normal life. He came off antidepressants and wrote an excellent book about depression, which he called *Malignant Sadness*.[8]

For nine years Mary was unable to eat in the company of any other human being, including her own children; she felt so unworthy. The only exception was if someone actually gave her the food. She had been an unhappy child, with an extremely judgmental mother. But her real depression began in her thirties when she split up from the father of her children. She stopped driving for fear of deliberately crashing the car. She couldn't concentrate and was found wandering the streets, lost. She describes her feelings as a terrifying emptiness. "It felt I was being destroyed bit by bit by a virus that would never go away. I was disappearing."

When she went to her general practitioner, she was always in floods of tears, but all the GP provided was Prozac. This helped a bit, but her mood remained dreadful for nine years.

Eventually, she decided to refer herself for psychological therapy. It was CBT. At first she was pessimistic about whether it could help. But halfway through her eleven weekly sessions it began to click. There were three things, she says, that helped most. One was a systematic analysis of her thoughts, which showed how unreasonably self-critical they were. The second was a daily written plan for positive actions and a daily record of things she was grateful for. And the third was behavioral experiments—such as eating in public bit by bit—within the safe context of therapy.

As a result her mood changed completely. She became a different person and has remained so for over four years.

Sophie is a beautiful, talented woman in her late twenties. She always suffered from perfectionism, and could never do as well as she thought she should. This made her unnaturally detached as a teenager, and at fifteen she was in a serious accident—not caring, it seemed, whether she survived. Academically, she flew high, and it was not till her last year at university that she really crashed.

She couldn't think straight and couldn't cope. She felt trapped, numb. She alternated between total emptiness and the frantic feeling of thoughts whirling out of control. She had an overwhelming desire to escape the horror of it all. In her room in the middle of the night she drank the whiskey and took the pills. Fortunately she was sick, and survived to complete her degree.

But the next year was worse than the one before. She quit her job and was in and out of work, unable to hold anything down. She was drinking a lot. She saw a counselor but it made little difference. Then she got referred for CBT.

She learned to observe and record her thoughts, which brought some calm; she became able to observe her perfectionism. She was also taught to schedule her life (her eating, sleeping, socializing, drinking), which brought order out of chaos. She went back to work. Bit by bit her mood lifted, and now she has been calm and stable for over two years. "I like myself more," she says, "and everybody notices the difference."

We all feel down at times, especially if something bad has happened to us. That is not what we mean here by depression. Depression may be triggered by an external event, but it is a feeling of overwhelming despair that persists much longer than normal unhappiness. Quite often there is no obvious trigger. In the words of the poet Coleridge,

A grief without a pang, void, dark, and drear,
A stifled, drowsy, unimpassioned grief,
Which finds no natural outlet, no relief,
In word, or sigh, or tear [9]

There are of course degrees of depression. [10] The formal definition of a major depression used by the American

Psychiatric Association[11] says that for at least two weeks you have experienced depressed mood for most of the time, and/ or lost interest and pleasure in nearly all activities. In addition you experienced at least three of the following almost every day:[12] reduced or increased sleep, reduced or increased weight, physical agitation or torpor, fatigue, loss of concentration, a sense of worthlessness, and suicidal thoughts. These must be bad enough to cause significant impairment in your normal functioning at home or at work almost every day. At any one time about 4% of adults in most advanced countries have a major depression, but another 4% or so have less severe depression—making 8% in all.

Table 2.1 shows the Patient Health Questionnaire (PHQ-9), whose nine questions are used as a screening device for depression. Table 2.2 shows the Generalized Anxiety Disorder questionnaire (GAD-7) used to screen for anxiety. When the depression scores are computed, this is how they are classified: 10–14 is called "Mild," 15–19 is "Moderate," and 20+ is "Severe." There are about equal numbers of depressed people in each of these three groups, and most major depressions score above 15.[13] As for anxiety, a score of 8 or more on the GAD-7 indicates a disorder.

To see how these scores change during therapy, we can look at Mary's experience (figure 2.1). She began with high levels of depression and anxiety. Halfway through she was down to the borderline level of disorder, and by the end she had hardly any remaining symptoms.

Depression tends to start at older ages than anxiety.[14] It rarely begins until the teens, and the average age of onset is thirty. And, unlike anxiety, depression tends to recur. Episodes mostly end within nine months, but among people who ex-

Table 2.1. PHQ-9 for depression

Over the last 2 weeks, how often have you been bothered by any of the following problems?	Not at all	Several days	More than half the days	Nearly every day
1. Little interest or pleasure in doing things	0	1	2	3
2. Feeling down, depressed, or hopeless	0	1	2	3
3. Trouble falling or staying asleep, or sleeping too much	0	1	2	3
4. Feeling tired or having little energy	0	1	2	3
5. Poor appetite or overeating	0	1	2	3
6. Feeling bad about yourself—or that you are a failure or have let yourself or your family down	0	1	2	3
7. Trouble concentrating on things, such as reading the newspaper or watching television	0	1	2	3
8. Moving or speaking so slowly that other people could have noticed? Or the opposite—being so fidgety or restless that you have been moving around a lot more than usual	0	1	2	3
9. Thoughts that you would be better off dead or of hurting yourself in some way	0	1	2	3

perience one episode, some 60% will have at least one more episode, and on average they will experience four episodes altogether during their life.[15] Some depressions are so serious that the person has to go to the hospital because they cannot cope at all or are in danger of killing themselves.

Hospitalization is particularly common among those people who sometimes experience depression but also at other times experience mania (excessive excitement, grandiosity, aggression, or lack of sleep). These people have an enduring

Table 2.2. GAD-7 for anxiety disorder

Over the last 2 weeks, how often have you been bothered by the following problems?	Not at all	Several days	More than half the days	Nearly every day
1. Feeling nervous, anxious, or on edge	0	1	2	3
2. Not being able to stop or control worrying	0	1	2	3
3. Worrying too much about different things	0	1	2	3
4. Trouble relaxing	0	1	2	3
5. Being so restless that it is	0	1	2	3
6. Becoming easily annoyed	0	1	2	3
7. Feeling afraid as if something	0	1	2	3

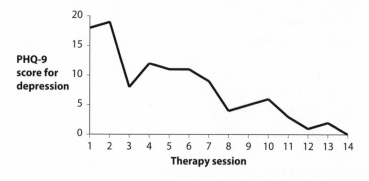

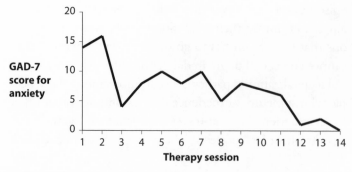

Figure 2.1. Mary's scores during treatment.

state called bipolar disorder, which generally emerges in the late teens or soon after.[16] This condition is generally more serious than unipolar depression (where there are no periods of mania). More than 10% of people with bipolar disorder eventually kill themselves.[17] Bipolar disorder affects about 0.5 to 1% of adults at any one time[18] and is one of the three main conditions known as "severe mental illness." The others are schizophrenia and personality disorder.

Schizophrenia

Schizophrenia can take many forms.[19] Deluded beliefs or hallucinations are the most common. Some deluded people believe they are someone else—God or the Devil or the President—generally *folies de grandeur*. Others believe they are the victims of persecution. By contrast, hallucinations are physical experiences—most commonly voices endlessly talking to them, or sometimes visions. We have all seen tragic figures in the street, engaged in furious argument with their voices, or denouncing an imagined outrage.

In all these cases schizophrenia has taken a "positive" form—with strange beliefs or experiences acted out. By contrast, roughly a quarter of people with schizophrenia are quite passive—apathetic, without pleasure or apparent emotion; they suffer but they suffer in silence. A third variety of symptom is disordered behavior—people's speech may be chaotic, they can laugh or cry wildly, or they may be catatonically immobile.

Schizophrenia is a strange and awful collection of conditions, well described in Sebastian Faulks's novel *Human Traces*. For relatives it is deeply disturbing. Schizophrenia is the most common form of "psychosis," meaning that in its acute phases the person is seriously out of contact with reality. About 10% of people with schizophrenia kill themselves.[20] The problem affects 0.5 to 1% of the population in most countries in the world and does not fully emerge until the late teens or later. More than 20% of people who have schizophrenia fully recover.[21]

Personality Disorder

People with personality disorder include two main groups.[22] The first are people with highly unstable lives and feelings. Many of them self-harm, and up to 10% eventually commit suicide. Their condition is known, somewhat oddly, as borderline personality disorder, and it affects 0.5 to 1% of the adult population.

The second group has antisocial personality disorder. These people regularly violate the normal rights of other people. They are often charming, and many of them are psychopathic in the sense that they have no sense of guilt and no remorse. They comprise another 0.5 to 1% of the adult population. Like people with borderline personality disorder, more than a third of them are substance abusers,[23] which tells us that inside they are not stable or happy.

Alcoholism and Drug Addiction

Dependence on alcohol or drugs can ruin many people's lives—and the lives of their families. Most of those who are seriously addicted also suffer from one of the conditions we have already discussed.[24] But one natural question is, which problem comes first? Did the addiction cause the depression/anxiety, or vice versa? To answer such a question, one would need detailed month-by-month histories of people to see what preceded what, and even then it could still be that some third factor caused both sets of problems.[25] But in practice it matters little which diagnosis is primary since generally it is essential to treat both sets of problems in parallel.

In the United States 1% of adults are deemed to be dependent on alcohol.[26] This is an alarming number, especially when so many alcoholics die of liver disease or suicide.[27] Some 18% of all people with severe alcoholism eventually commit suicide, typically after twenty years or more of heavy drinking.[28]

Hard drugs like cocaine and heroin are a somewhat smaller social problem than alcohol, but again the results are often tragic. Accidental death is not uncommon. In the United States about 0.5% of adults are dependent on hard drugs. These are the people known as "problem drug users." The majority have mental health problems,[29] and many have alcohol problems also.

A final form of addiction is gambling. Something like 0.3% of adults are pathological gamblers—mostly men. Gambling, like all addiction, is most common in early adulthood and falls steadily with age.[30]

Indeed, many of the problems we have been discussing begin in childhood, and half of all those who experience mental illness as adults already showed serious mental health problems before they were fifteen.[31] Child mental illness not only blights childhood but more often than not also leads on to adult mental illness.

Troubled Children

Brian is a neat, polite boy, age eight. But he was not always nice. From eighteen months on he had temper tantrums, often four times a day. He would smash things, attack his mother with knives, steal her money, and threaten to jump from the balcony of their apartment. His charming mother has had cervical cancer since Brian was born. Yet on one occasion he deliberately kicked her on the wound just after she had an operation. The wound split open and the operation had to be repeated.

At school Brian was equally restless, constantly roaming the classroom; he was repeatedly sent out for disruptive behavior. He had no friends because he was so aggressive. By the age of six he was out of control, and his mother was discussing with social services whether he could be taken into care.

Instead, by great good luck, he was referred for specialist help to a leading psychiatric clinic. He was diagnosed with oppositional defiant disorder. Brian and his mother then met each week with a senior psychiatrist to play the "parent-child game," where the psychiatrist teaches the parent how to appreciate and praise the child wherever possible. At once Brian began to improve—his mother was a good learner. But Brian was still restless. So he was assessed for attention deficit hyperactivity disorder (ADHD) and found to have it. He was therefore also put on a daily dose of medication.

Within two months of starting at the clinic, Brian was quite a different person. He was calm most of the time, and when he wasn't, he knew to take himself off to his room to calm down. Tantrums declined to once every two months, rather than four times a day. He was never again excluded from classes, and he became affectionate to his mother. Two years on, he is still doing just fine.

At any one time some 10% of children have a diagnosable mental disorder.[32] Roughly 3% suffer from an anxiety disorder, such as social phobia, which can undermine learning and lead them to leave school early.[33] Fewer have depression, which even by early adolescence only affects just over 1%.

More suffer from conduct disorder, like Brian's. It affects some 5% of all children at any one time. A child who is out of control before the age of ten is highly likely to become a badly behaved or criminal adult later on.[34] By comparison, other young people who only become impossible as teenagers are much less likely to persist with bad behavior into adulthood.

Some children have ADHD. They are inattentive, and often hyperactive and impulsive in their behavior. ADHD generally reveals itself by the age of four. It affects 1–2% of children, and the majority of them also in due course exhibit conduct disorder.[35]

Children with autism compose the most tragic group. As always, there is a spectrum of severity, with roughly one in 150 children affected in some way. These children lack the normal ability to understand other people's meanings and other people's feelings. They make no eye contact and communicate poorly. A third of them never learn to speak, but others can, with help, become functioning and independent adults.

Mental and Physical Pain

All the problems we have discussed in this chapter involve pain—pain of the mind. Mental pain is as real as physical pain, and indeed the emotional aspect of physical pain is experienced in exactly the same brain areas as mental pain (the anterior cingulate cortex and anterior insula).[36] It is no surprise that we use the same word to describe both mental and physical pain. In fact we almost always use the same words for both. We can have a "hurt" foot or "hurt" feelings, we can have toothache or heartache, and we can have physical illness or mental illness.

But we have to be careful with the phrase "mental illness." In clinical practice one would never use it; one would talk about mental health problems or difficulties. But where the issue is about policy and the spending of money, different language helps. Everybody has mental health problems of some sort, so if it is a contest between physical illness and "mental health problems," mental health often loses out. To make sure that people who need treatment get it, it helps to use the concept of mental illness. This absolutely does not imply that their problem is biological, but simply that they have a clinical condition that needs treatment. The same is true if they have broken their leg on the football field—the cause of their problem is not biological but they need treatment. There are many terms to describe the psychological disorders we are discussing, and we deliberately use different phrases at different points in the book.

Since we all have problems, we all lie at some point on a spectrum of mental health. So there is an issue about where to draw the borderline between those who are ill and those who are not. But this is no different from the case with many physical illnesses. For example, what is "high blood pressure"? The answer is that clinicians look at the way blood pressure affects the probability of heart attack and say that blood pressure is high when it raises the probability of heart attack by an unacceptable amount. The same is true of mental illness. The cutoff is where the level of distress is unacceptably high or the condition interferes unacceptably with a person's life.

And what about the concept of diagnosis? Some people dislike it on the grounds that it "medicalizes" mental illness and that people often have a whole range of problems. But if we want to help people, we must be able to identify their central problem and then use whatever treatment has been found to help other people with the same problem. This is not a "medical model." It is the same scientific model that is applied to solving any problem, be it social, psychological, biological, or mechanical. And, interestingly, diagnosis can be more valuable in guiding psychological treatments than drug treatments. Essentially the same antidepressants are likely to be prescribed for depression and most of the different anxiety disorders, but there are major differences in the way psychological treatments are applied to those conditions.

There are of course many types of mental disorder, and there is no imperative need for a single encompassing definition (any more than there is for a single definition of physical illness). But a good enough definition of mental illness is "significant and persistent distress and impairment of functioning, with causes that are psychological or psychophysical." This definition of course includes senile dementia.

But we shall not cover that since it is a very discrete problem coming at the end of life,[37] and the illnesses discussed in this chapter are already enough for one book.

Our central focus is on the millions who suffer from depression and anxiety disorders (and conduct disorder among children). Most of them are not in treatment (while most of those with severe mental illness are). Theirs is the central problem we address.

But just how many people do all these conditions affect? Is the situation getting worse? And how many are getting the treatment they need?

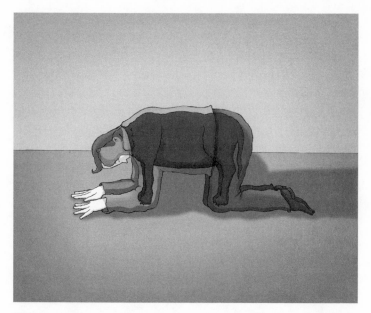

Black dog

3 * How Many Suffer?

Dr. Sillitoe's got him on tablets for depression. It's not mental, in fact it's quite widespread. A lot of better-class people get it apparently.

Alan Bennett, Enjoy

The scale of mental illness is mind-boggling. In table 3.1 we pull together the figures for the different conditions and see that altogether roughly one in five of all adults are suffering, and roughly one in ten of all children.

For adults, as for children, this figure excludes the mildest levels of disorder. If instead these are included, the figure becomes somewhat larger—26% in the United States, 23% in Britain, and 27% in the European Union.[1] But in the United States, for example, over a third of those included in the figure have "mild" conditions, while a third are "moderate," and under a third "severe."[2] To get a feel for what these definitions mean, we can ask for how long in the last year these people were unable to perform their normal role. For severe cases the average time "out of role" is over two months, but for mild ones it is under a day. So we prefer the somewhat narrower definition of the problem used in our table.

But is mental illness as common in poorer countries as it is in richer ones? On the available evidence, it is—for depression, anxiety, and schizophrenia. Table 3.2 gives the figures for depression (on a slightly narrower definition than the previous table).[3] Quite rightly, the World Health Organization repeatedly points out that mental ill health is a worldwide problem.[4]

Table 3.1. Percentage of people suffering from mental illness

Adults		Children (5–16)	
Anxiety disorders	8	Anxiety disorders	3
Depression	8	Depression	1
Schizophrenia and bipolar	1	Autistic spectrum disorder	1
Personality disorder	1	Conduct disorder/ADHD	5
Severe substance dependence	1		
Total	19	Total	10

Table 3.2. Percentage of adults suffering from depression

High-income countries	6.5
Upper-middle-income countries	5.5
Lower-middle-income countries	6.5
Low-income countries	7.0

All these figures relate to people who are ill at some point in time, or within some particular year. But there are also many others alive who are currently well but have been ill at some point, or will become so. In fact at least a third of the population will experience mental illness at some point in their lives.[5] Moreover, mental illness also affects the families of those who are ill. On a rough calculation, about 30% of all households now include one adult who is mentally ill[6]—and the figure would be even higher if we could also include households where a child is mentally ill.

Turning to children, mental illness is once again a world-wide problem. As figure 3.1 shows, mental illness is as common in the poorest countries as in the richest.[7]

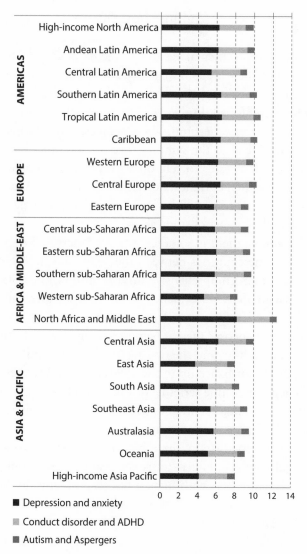

Figure 3.1. Prevalence of mental disorders among children under 19 (percentage).

Getting Worse?

Are there more mental health problems now than there used to be? There are some data that suggest that things have got much worse, and these findings have received a lot of publicity. But for adults these results are mostly based on retrospective survey questions, where people are asked whether they have ever had the symptoms of mental illness and at what age.[8] It is safer to rely on surveys where people are asked about their current state of mind, and the same survey is then repeated later with similar populations of people. What do these types of study show?

For adults, there is some evidence of increased depression in some countries between the 1950s and the 1990s.[9] But since then comprehensive surveys in the United States and Britain show no evidence of further increases among adults.[10] So there is no "epidemic of depression."

For young people there is better long-term evidence than there is for adults, and the findings are broadly similar—of increased disturbance up to the 1990s but stability thereafter. The longest time series is for four-year college students in the United States and goes back to the 1940s. Figure 3.2 shows the figures for depression.[11]

Similarly for Britain, there have been four comparable national surveys of fifteen- to sixteen-year-olds, beginning in 1974. The numbers with mental health problems doubled between 1974 and 1999, but were stable between then and 2004.[12] Another study of the same age group in Scotland alone showed similar increases in emotional problems up to 1999.[13] Interestingly, this increase affected all social classes and both sexes. Further questioning showed that the main causes were greater stress over relationships, body image, and exams.

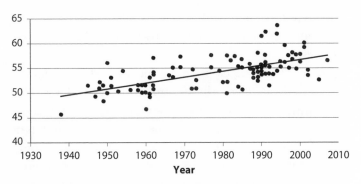

Figure 3.2. Depression scores of US college students have increased since the 1940s.

It seems possible that many conditions, especially depression, may now begin earlier in people's lives than they did thirty or forty years ago. However, the number of people affected at any stage in their lives has probably grown a lot less. Mental illnesses have been around since humans first evolved. What is new is that they can now be treated.

The Burden of Disease

It is natural to ask how common mental illness is, when compared with physical illness. We could of course simply compare the number of people who had each type of clinical condition. But this would fail to reflect the degree of pain caused by the different illnesses and the extent to which they interfere with normal living. For example, one World Health Organization (WHO) study compared the degree of disability caused by depression with that caused by four of the most common chronic physical illnesses—diabetes, angina, asthma, and arthritis. It found that depression is 50% more severe and disabling than any of the other four illnesses.[14]

The WHO has developed a specific methodology for evaluating the scale of morbidity caused by each illness. This takes the numbers with each illness and then weights them by the degree of disability each illness causes.[15] The results of their 2008 exercise are truly astonishing. In advanced countries, mental illness accounts for 38% of the total amount of morbidity.[16] This contrasts with 6% for cardiovascular disease and even less for diabetes. The numbers are shown in figure 3.3. Within mental illness, more than a half of the total is accounted for by depression and anxiety disorders.

In terms of morbidity, mental illness is the most common group of illnesses by far. But it is not an immediate cause of death (except in the case of suicide). To measure the "overall" burden of different diseases, we also have to take into account the premature deaths they cause. The WHO measures the burden of premature death by the years of life lost through death before the age of eighty. They then add to this

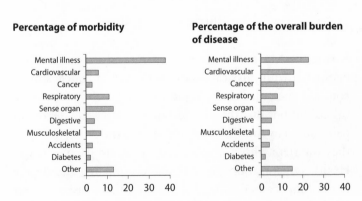

Figure 3.3. Mental illness is the biggest health problem in rich countries.

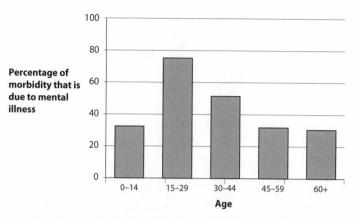

Figure 3.4. Mental illness is the main health problem of working age in rich countries.

burden the burden of morbidity, treating one year of morbidity as equivalent to the partial loss of a year of life. The result for advanced countries is shown in the right-hand graph in figure 3.3. It shows that, even when we allow for premature death, the burden of mental illness is still bigger than that of cardiovascular disease or cancer. In advanced countries it accounts for 23% of the overall burden of disease.

For the world as a whole, the overall figures are: mental health 13%, cardiovascular disease 10%, cancer 5%, respiratory diseases 4%, and diabetes 1%.[17] Yet when the United Nations decided to hold its first ever conference on noncommunicable diseases in 2011, it included all the last four diseases—but not mental illness.

This is particularly surprising since mental illness causes not only massive suffering but also great economic waste. This is because mental illness is especially a disease of working age. Figure 3.4 shows the percentage of morbidity caused by mental illness at each age. While physical illness is mainly a disease of old age,[18] mental illness accounts for over half of all illness up to age forty-five. It is by far the most important disease of working age.

Suicide

These facts should be enough to persuade people that mental illness is a much bigger problem than most policy makers allow for. But if not, the final argument comes from suicide.[19] About 90% of people who kill themselves are mentally ill when they do it.[20] Although half are also physically ill, it is the mental pain rather than the physical pain that generally drives people to take their lives. Suicide is rare among physically ill people who are not also mentally ill.[21]

As many people in the world die from suicide as from homicide and warfare combined. For example, in the year 2000, 815,000 people killed themselves while 520,000 people were murdered, and 310,000 died through war.[22] In most advanced countries between 0.5% and 2% of people end their lives by suicide, as figure 3.5 shows.

Which types of mental illness account for most of these suicides? In table 3.3 we take a representative country where 1% of deaths are by suicide. As the bottom row of the table shows, some 60% of those who kill themselves were suffering from unipolar depression, 10% from bipolar disorder, 10% from schizophrenia, and 10% from personality disorders. But unipolar depression is much more common in the population than the other conditions, so the individual's risk of suicide is much lower for people with unipolar

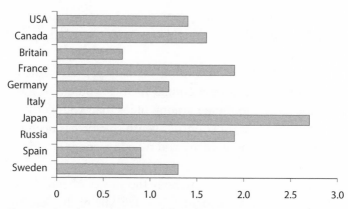

Figure 3.5. Suicide as a percentage of all deaths (latest year).

Table 3.3. Schematic map of lifetime suicide rates

	Depression excluding bipolar	Bipolar disorder	Schizophrenia	Personality disorder	None of these
(A) What % of people ever have this condition?	15%	1%	1%	2%	82%
(B) What % of these commit suicide?	4%	10%	10%	5%	0.1%
(C) What % of people ever have this condition and commit suicide? ((A)x(B))	0.6%	0.1%	0.1%	0.1%	0.1%

(*Note*: The total rate in Row C is 1%).

depression than it is for people with bipolar disorder or schizophrenia. Alcoholism is also a major contributing factor in many suicides.

In most countries, including the United States, suicide is over twice as common among men as women. In most countries it is also higher among older than younger people. However, in most countries youth suicide has been rising (especially among men), and suicide among the elderly has been falling.

Much has been written about the causes of suicide. In 1897 the French sociologist Émile Durkheim divided suicides into three groups: anomic (where society provides no clear sense of purpose), altruistic (where social pressure is excessive), and egoistic (where there was a personal history of social isolation, mental or physical illness, or bereavement). But Durkheim stressed in particular the first two social factors. He was partly right. As we shall see in chapter 7, there are important social factors that explain the different prevalence of misery in differing societies. There are also technical factors like the availability of firearms or unfenced bridges. But to explain who commits suicide in a given society, we need to focus on the differences between individuals.

Why is suicide so heavily male? And why do some mentally ill people commit suicide while most do not? The best predictor of suicide is hopelessness—a feeling that there is no way out. Suffering can be borne if you can see light at the end of the tunnel. But if there is no hope, why go on? Yet even then some extra element is needed—enough energy to do the deed. So the second predictor of successful suicide is impulsiveness, which is much more common among men than women. The lethal combination is an impulsive personality, low in self-esteem, and an intolerable external situation involving bullying, rejection, or failure.[23]

Many suicides are highly impulsive: two-thirds of unsuccessful suicide attempts were not envisaged an hour before the attempt.[24] Others are much more planned, especially those 30% of successful suicides where a suicide note is left.

Winston Churchill was an impulsive man with a strong depressive element in his character, which he called his black dog.[25] Here is what he wrote about suicide:

> I don't like standing near the edge of a platform when an express train is passing through. I like to stand right back and if possible get a pillar between me and the train. I don't like to stand by the side of a ship and look down into the water. A second's action would end everything. A few drops of desperation.

Thankfully there are a huge number of suicide attempts that do not succeed. Thus in Britain in any particular year 0.7% of people attempt suicide and fail.[26] About 5% of adults say they have attempted suicide at some point in their lives.[27] Unsuccessful suicide attempts have a very different pattern from successful ones. They are more common among women than men, by a ratio of at least 2:1. And they are much more common among young people than older people. Moreover, while only about 20% of successful suicides are by taking an overdose, around 90% of unsuccessful attempts are.

This does not mean that an unsuccessful suicide attempt is just a cry for help. It is a cry of pain and entrapment.[28] As the psychologist Mark Williams of Oxford University puts it, a bird defeated in battle by another bird tends to fly away, if it can. But if it is trapped with the other bird in a cage, it just crumples up and wastes away. People who attempt suicide often do not care whether they live or die; they simply leave it to chance.[29]

Mental health is a huge humanitarian issue—a massive cause of suffering and disability. But do those who need help get it?

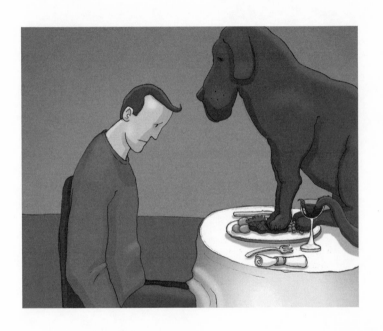

4 * Do They Get Help?

My daughter Charlotte suffers from depression
associated with OCD, and she attempted suicide two
weeks ago (it was a serious attempt). But she is still not
in treatment despite being referred ten months ago.
If she had a physical illness equivalent to this mental
illness she is battling with, she would have been rushed
to hospital, and appropriate treatment would have been
forthcoming.

Letter to Richard Layard, May 2009

The scale of mental illness may be mind-boggling, but what
is really shocking is the lack of help. Although, as we shall
see, really effective treatments exist, most people get no help
at all.

The Scandal of Undertreatment

The contrast with physical illness is striking. In rich countries over 90% of people with diabetes are in treatment. But
most people with mental illnesses are not. In the United
States, Britain, and continental Europe, fewer than a third
are in treatment. Even for major depression the figure is
under half.[1] The situation is even worse in low- and middle-
income countries where, as table 4.1 shows, fewer than 10%
of people with mental illness are in treatment.[2]

In most countries the main form of treatment is medication. For example, in 2007, 15% of British adults with
anxiety or depression were getting just medication, while

Table 4.1. Percentage of adult sufferers who get treated

United States	33%
Britain	31%
European Union	26%
Low and middle-income countries	9%

only 10% were getting any form of face-to-face therapy or counseling (with or without medication).[3] But national treatment guidelines say that 100% should be offered some form of psychological therapy and many fewer should be offered medication.

Figure 4.1 shows the treatment rates in Britain for different conditions.[4] For children the situation is as dire as it is for adults: only a quarter are in treatment.[5]

How long do people have these problems until they get treated? Many people with mental disorders never get treated. Even thirty years after their social phobia first began, 70% of people in the United States have never been treated, nor have 25% of people with depression. For people who do get treated, the average time they wait is sixteen years for social phobia, nine years for generalized anxiety, and eight years for depression. Even for bipolar disorder it is six years.[6] Strikingly, only 28% of suicides in Britain had been in contact with mental health services in the previous twelve months.[7]

Of course many of these people never asked for treatment. But those who do often face intolerable waits. This would be a shocking situation if it applied to a condition that is rare. It is even more shocking when it applies to one of the most serious and most common of all health problems.

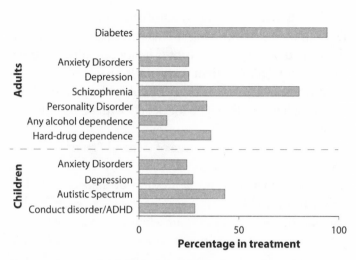

Figure 4.1. Most mental illness goes untreated.
The treatment rates are for Britain in 2007 except for the diabetes figure which is for high-income countries as a whole.

Rationing

Why are so few people in treatment? The immediate reason is without doubt the underprovision of psychological therapy. Almost anyone who is mentally ill can get pills from their GP. But most people want more than this—they want help in managing their mental life. They want an explanation of what is going on, and many want a diagnosis. Medication on its own provides none of this, and it can also have unpleasant side effects that discourage people from seeking or continuing treatment. Three-quarters of patients who go to the doctor with mental health problems want psychological therapy,[8] and most cannot get what they need.

There is overwhelming evidence of the rationing of mental health services involving specialist psychological care. In the United States two-thirds of primary care physicians say they cannot get outpatient services for people with mental health problems; this is at least double the number who have problems finding help for people with physical health problems.[9]

In Britain the Royal College of General Practitioners did a survey of its members in 2010. They were asked, "When adults are suffering from depression or anxiety disorders requiring specialist psychological therapy, e.g., cognitive behavioral therapy (not just counseling), are you able to get them this treatment within two months?," followed by a similar question about children with emotional or behavioral problems. Only 15% of the GPs who responded said they could usually get the adult service needed, and 65% said they could rarely get it. For children the results were even worse, with only 6% usually able to get the service and 78% rarely able to do so.[10]

In the short term the blame rests firmly on those who fund the provision of psychological therapy—in the United States and many other countries insurers, and in Britain the local commissioners in the National Health Service. Nearly all systems ration psychological care in a way they would not consider for physical illnesses of comparable severity. For example, many will only pay for six sessions of therapy—as if it might be all right to authorize half a heart operation.

By contrast medication is readily available. The contrast is striking. Medication resembles the way in which doctors treat other diseases and is therefore something they can understand. Very few general practitioners (some of them wonderful) have had any significant period of training in common mental disorders, even though these account for some 25% of the time they spend with patients. Secondly, medication is produced by drug companies, who are very effective at lobbying. There is no equivalent lobbying for psychological therapy, even though that is what the majority of patients want. This brings us close to the main underlying explanation of the present situation: stigma.[11]

Stigma

People who are depressed or hyper-anxious are ashamed of themselves, while people with a broken leg or a heart condition are not. Mental illness makes you feel you have a fundamental flaw, which you do your best to hide. You may not even admit it to your friends or relatives, still less go to the doctor. And if you do, you are less likely to insist that the doctor find a solution. Your family also is ashamed, and usually creates little fuss. It is bad enough to feel terrible, but it is even worse if you cannot talk about it because you are so ashamed. Some people take their lives, but many more live on in pain, made worse by concealment.

And here is a second reason. Many people think that mental illness is untreatable, or that at best you can be helped to manage your condition. They do not realize that, with proper help, most people can recover. This issue is vital, and even now too many people in the mental health field talk of how their patients need to be supported, rather than cured. When the public thinks little can be done about something, they avoid talking about it. They ask people with physical illnesses how they are doing, but they avoid asking the same of people with mental illness. This merely reinforces the shame.

But there is hope. When cancer was largely untreatable, people hid it. Only as it has become treatable have people talked about their condition. And the fear and dread have been greatly reduced. Likewise, as more and more disabilities have become treatable, people have become much more open and straightforward about their disability. So have their families. And they have often formed themselves into extremely effective lobby groups. The same needs to happen with mental illness.

Conversations about mental illness will always of course involve one basic problem—it is difficult for other people to know just how ill you are. This applies somewhat to any illness, since all pain is subjective and other people can only infer how bad it is. But the problem is especially bad with mental health, since it is closely tied to how a person behaves.

Society works because we normally treat people as if they are responsible for their actions—as if they had free will. If they don't get up in the morning, we behave as if they could and we harass them until they do.

But of course sometimes they can't get up. If their leg is broken, it's quite obvious that they can't. But if they are in a major depression, it's less obvious whether they could get up or not. Quite possibly they simply couldn't. But if other people don't know enough about mental illness, they simply don't know how they should treat people with mental health problems. This is true within the family, and it is also true in schools and at work.

Obviously the answer is for everyone to know more about mental illness and to recognize when people can't do quite normal things unless they get help. The object of such help is of course to enable people to help themselves—to become once more responsible for what they do. But a key first step is to be able to ask, "Are you OK?"—to recognize that people may need help.

We are much more likely to ask this if we also know what to do if they say, "No, I'm not OK." This means that everyone has got to become more mental health conscious, better informed about what treatments exist, and more confident that recovery is possible.

So the way forward is clear.

- Everyone needs some training in mental health and in the possibilities of recovery—be they parents, teachers, employers, or health workers.
- People who care about this issue need to organize and campaign for better treatment—as people with physical disabilities and physical illnesses have done. Antistigma campaigns are a useful part of this.[12]
- And anyone who has a mental health problem should be as open about it as they can possibly be.

Heroes and Heroines

This is particularly true if they are in the public eye. We have seen how well-known figures who are homosexual have totally transformed public attitudes by coming out. The same will be true in mental health. So we should salute any well-known figure who has the guts to admit to a problem with their mental health.

We should salute the Norwegian prime minister, Kjell-Magne Bondevik, who took a month off for depression in 1998 and returned to win the next general election. We should salute Britain's former deputy prime minister, John Prescott, who has spoken publicly of his battle with bulimia. We should salute sports stars like the Olympic swimmer Michael Phelps (ADHD) and the England soccer player David Beckham (OCD). And TV personalities like John Madden (phobia), Stephen Fry (bipolar), or Ruby Wax (depression). And the popular author Marian Keyes (depression) and the actress Angelina Jolie (self-harm).

Marcus Trescothick is a great English cricketer whose international career was cut short by depression. In 2008 he came out in his book *Coming Back to Me*. The response astonished him. There was no stigma, only sympathy and support: "The impact of it was so completely different to what I expected."

In 2012 the British Parliament had a debate on mental health. It was known that 19% of British Members of Parliament had had problems with mental health at some period in their lives,[13] yet none had spoken about it. But in this debate no less than four Members of Parliament revealed the awful truth.[14] One had had major depression, one still has obsessive-compulsive disorder after thirty-one years, and two had had postnatal depression and panic attacks.

This is how Andrea Leadsom described her postnatal depression: "It is unbelievable how awful you feel when you are sitting with your tiny baby in your arms and your baby cries, and so do you. You cannot even make yourself a cup of tea. You just feel so utterly useless."

Charles Walker spoke of his OCD:

Over the past thirty-one years OCD has played a fairly significant part in my life. On occasions it is manageable and on occasions it becomes quite difficult. It takes one to some quite dark places. I operate to the rule of four, so I have to do everything in evens. I have to wash my hands four times and I have to go in and out of a room four times. My wife and children often say I resemble an extra from *Riverdance* as I bounce in and out of a room, switching lights off four times. Woe betide me if I switch off a light five times because then I have to do it another three times. Counting becomes very important. I leave cracker and cookie packets around the house because if I go near a bin, I have to wash my hands on numerous occasions.

OCD is like someone inside one's head banging away. One is constantly striking deals with oneself. Sometimes these are quite ridiculous and on some occasions they can be rather depressing and serious. I have been pretty healthy for five years, but just when you let your guard down, this aggressive friend comes and smacks you right in the face. I was on holiday recently and I took a beautiful photograph of my son carrying a fishing rod. I was glowing with pride and then the voice started, "If you don't get rid of that photograph, your child will die." You fight those voices for a couple or three hours, and you know that you really should not give in to them because they should not be there and it ain't going to happen. But in the end, you ain't going to risk your child, so one gives in to the voices and then feels pretty miserable about life.

These were brave men and women who spoke up. But in all four cases it appears that their reputations were improved by the courage they had shown. Kevan Jones, who had suffered from depression, admitted that before the debate he had still not decided whether to speak up. But he did, and this is how he ended: "I do not know whether I have done the right thing. Perhaps I will go home tonight and think I have not, but I think I have. I hope that it does not change anyone's view of me." It did—for the better.

An effective campaign for mental health requires personal testimony. But it also needs systematic information on how mental illness affects every aspect of life.

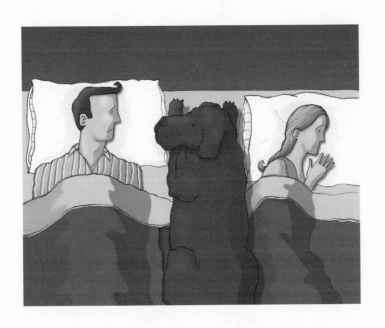

5 * How Does It Affect People's Lives?

Man delights not me; no, nor woman neither

Hamlet, *Act II, Scene ii*

Mental illness causes intense misery. In fact it is the biggest single cause of misery in modern societies. And it does a lot else to people's lives. Here are some of the extraordinary facts we shall explore:

- Mental illness causes more of the suffering in our society than physical illness does, or than poverty or unemployment do.
- It reduces life expectancy as much as smoking does.
- It accounts for nearly half of all the disabled people on disability benefits, and nearly half of all days off sick.
- It affects educational achievement and income as much as pure IQ does.

Suffering

We can begin with suffering. Until recently there was no way of examining scientifically what factors are really important for happiness and misery. But the new science of happiness is changing all that. People can now be asked how satisfied they are with their life, on a scale such as 0 (not at all satisfied) to 10 (very satisfied), and their answers are found to correlate well with objective measurements in the relevant parts of the brain.[1] So policy makers can increasingly design their policies to maximize the life-satisfaction of the population, rather than, for example, the level of national income.

To do this, we need to know what factors affect life-satisfaction and by how much. Surveys of the population help us here. These surveys reveal the huge impact of people's mental health but also of their physical health, income, work, family situation, age, and gender. These analyses have been done on many surveys in many countries with very similar results.[2]

In each case we look at who is miserable (that is, the lowest in terms of life-satisfaction). We then ask who these unhappy people are. How many are unemployed or poor (in the bottom 10% of income per head). How many are physically ill (in the bottom 10% of physical health). And how many have been diagnosed for depression or anxiety?

As figure 5.1 shows, the answer is remarkable. More of the most miserable people are suffering from diagnosed depression or anxiety disorders than from physical illness. And more are suffering from depression or anxiety disorders than from either poverty or unemployment. The diagram is for the United States, but the position is similar in Britain, Germany, and Australia. However one does the analysis, mental illness emerges as the biggest single factor affecting whether someone is not satisfied with their life.[3]

The result is striking. Crucially, *mental ill health explains more of the misery in the population than physical illness does.* This is so, even though we are looking at all age groups including the elderly, for whom physical health can be a real problem. And mental ill health also explains a lot more misery than is explained by poverty or by unemployment.

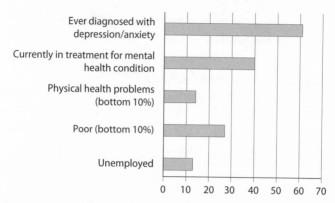

Figure 5.1. Percentage of those in misery having each characteristic. Misery is the bottom 5.6% of life-satisfaction.

So we really need a new concept of deprivation, which includes much more than material poverty. Whatever financial means you have, you are deeply deprived if you do not have the psychological means to enjoy your life. Public policy needs to put mental health much nearer the center stage.

Mental health should be put equal to physical health. To see why, we can observe that health impacts on five main dimensions of people's lives—their physical mobility, their ability to care for themselves, their ability to do their usual activities, their physical pain, and their mental pain. We can then ask which of these dimensions has the biggest effect on a person's satisfaction with life. The following analysis gives the results for a representative sample of US citizens.[4] As figure 5.2 shows, mental pain has a bigger negative effect than physical pain. One reason is that it is less easy to adapt to. While it is possible to think about other things than one's physical pain, mental pain has a horrible tendency to occupy the whole space of consciousness.

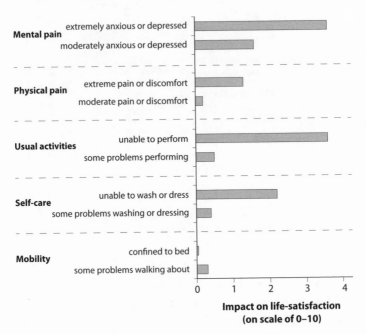

Figure 5.2. How much do different dimensions of illness reduce life-satisfaction?

Unfortunately, people who have not been mentally ill cannot easily imagine how awful it is. Thus when the public is asked to rate the five dimensions in order of importance, they rate mental pain as no worse than physical pain or physical immobility.[5] Yet for those who experience it, mental illness is in fact worse than most physical illness.

Sickness and Death

Mental illness also has a major effect on your physical health. The mind affects the body (and vice versa). So here is another extraordinary fact. *Depression has the same effect on life expectancy as smoking does*—and not mainly through suicide. For example, one study covered everybody in the Norwegian county of Nord-Trøndelag. At the beginning of the study they all received a clinical diagnosis of their mental state. They were then followed for up to six years to see who died. It was found that, at any particular age, you were 52% more likely to die if you were originally depressed than if you were not.[6] This was almost exactly the same difference in death rate as between those who were smokers when interviewed and those who were not.

Other studies have found similar results in the United States and Britain. One study focused simply on people's happiness (measured by a few simple questions).[7] They interviewed a sample of British people aged over fifty and then followed them for the next nine years, recording whether they had died. Those who were least happy to begin with were the most likely to die. Indeed, as figure 5.3 shows, the differences were very striking. And even after controlling for age and any illnesses they already had, people in the least

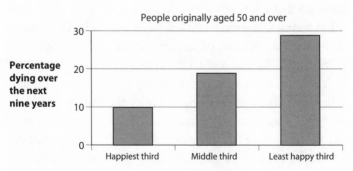

Figure 5.3. Unhappy people are more likely to die.

happy group were 50% more likely to die each year than people in the happiest group.[8]

But what diseases are they more likely to die of? We know more about the effects of depression than of anxiety, and depression seems to increase the risk of most forms of chronic illness. A sample survey of Canadian adults in 1994 distinguished between those experiencing major depression in that year and the rest of the population. It then followed both groups over the following eight years to see what new diseases they developed. Controlling for age and sex, the depressed people were at least 50% more likely to develop heart disease, stroke, lung disease, asthma, and arthritis.[9] Similarly in a meta-analysis focused on cancer, people with stress-related psychological problems were more likely to develop the disease.[10]

Moreover, mental illness also affects the progress of a physical disease once it has begun. To show this, we have to be careful to control for the initial severity of the physical illness. But when we have done this, we still find that mental illness has an important effect on what happens. For patients with cancer, a review of twenty-five studies shows that on average patients who have major or minor depression are up to 40% more likely to die each year.[11] And for people who have had a heart attack, the chances of dying are 50% higher among those with depression or anxiety disorders.[12] The figure of "50% more likely to die" seems to be a recurring theme.

There are many reasons for this.[13] First, if a person is mentally ill doctors are less likely to notice the physical illness.[14] So undertreatment is one reason. Second, some psychiatric medications have bad physical side effects. Third, mentally ill people often lead more unhealthy lives—they smoke and drink more, take more drugs, eat worse, and exercise less.[15]

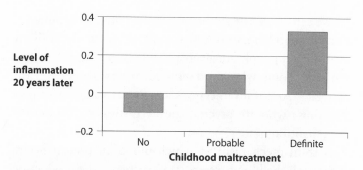

Figure 5.4. Child maltreatment affects inflammation 20 years later. Inflammation is a composite measure based on C-reactive protein, fibrinogen, and white blood cell count. It is standardized to mean 0 and SD = 1.

But the main reason is probably the direct effect of chronic stress upon the body. *Chronic stress damages the body in many ways.*[16] First, it leads to constant activation of the fight-or-flight response. This involves over-production of the hormone adrenaline, and abnormal patterns of the hormone cortisol.[17] The result is shorter life expectancy. Stress also triggers chronic general inflammation with detrimental health consequences, such as furring of the arteries and insulin resistance. For example, a study of children born in Dunedin, New Zealand, showed a powerful link between child abuse in the first ten years of life and the level of inflammation biomarkers twenty years later. This is illustrated in figure 5.4.[18]

Another study looked at the effects of psychological trauma occurring when you are an adult. A random sample was taken of all those who served in the US army in Vietnam. Some seventeen years later they were given a medical examination. Those veterans who had got chronic post-traumatic stress disorder were three times more likely than others to have auto-immune diseases (such as rheumatoid arthritis, type-1 diabetes, or psoriasis).[19]

We can also verify the effect of mood on the immune system through laboratory experiments. Here are two striking examples. If people are given a standard small experimental wound, people who are depressed or anxious recover the slowest.[20] And if flu injections are given to a group of people, those who are psychologically distressed develop the fewest antibodies.[21]

A third mechanism by which mood affects our health is through the bloodstream: stress increases the production of fibrinogen and the adhesiveness of platelets. These make blood clots and heart attacks more likely.[22]

Through all these mechanisms mental stress produces physical symptoms by affecting the organic state of the body. But sometimes there is also a different mechanism. This is where people experience bodily symptoms but doctors can find no corresponding organic disorder—the so-called medically unexplained symptoms. The symptoms are real enough: the person feels back pain, abdominal pain, chest pain, headache, or whatever, but no organic cause can be discovered or treated. This is extremely common. Believe it or not, in the outpatient clinics of two large South London hospitals, half of all the patients referred to them have medically unexplained symptoms.[23] In some of these cases there are doubtless organic disorders that the doctors cannot detect, but in the other cases the very real symptoms are caused directly by the person's mental state. In all these cases psychological treatments may be useful.

Two millennia ago, the great Greco-Roman doctor Galen opined that 60% of patients visiting the doctor had symptoms that had emotional rather than physical causes.[24] This was probably an overestimate, but there are certainly powerful links running from mind to body, which we have traced in this chapter. There are also of course links in the opposite direction—from body to mind:[25] if you have a chronic physical illness, you are roughly three times more likely to be depressed or hyper-anxious.[26] But this is for chapter 7.

It is enough to say here that one way to improve physical health is through better mental health. When the Romans idolized "the healthy mind in the healthy body," they meant that each supports the other. If only more doctors thought like that today.

Inability to Work

If mental health problems can damage your physical health, they can also stop you working. Indeed some of this effect comes about indirectly through physical disease. But even if we ignore the effect on physical health, over a third of all disability comes directly from mental illness. This is true in the United States, Britain, and continental Europe—as table 5.1, the numbers on disability benefits, shows. Altogether, roughly 6% of working-age adults are on disability benefits, and over a third of these are there for explicit reasons of mental illness. On top of this many people who report physical illness, like back pain or headache, have medically unexplained symptoms that are psychosomatic in origin. So close to 50% of disability benefits are directly due to mental illness.

One reason for the high number on welfare is that if you get on welfare due to mental illness, you are likely to stay there for a long time. In Britain the average time is four years. The shocking thing is that, even when people are drawing taxpayers' money because of their mental illness, under

Table 5.1. What percentage of people of working age are on disability benefits?

	Due to all causes	Due to mental illness
United States	6.6	2.0
Britain	6.1	2.5
6 other OECD countries (av)	6.4	2.4

Table 5.2. Percentage of potential working days lost through sickness absence

	% for workers with mental illness	% for all other workers
Britain	11.0	2.2
21 European countries	11.2	4.6

half of them (in Britain at least) are in any form of treatment.[27] That is not good for anybody.

Moreover, even if you have a job, mental health problems make it harder to perform well. Mentally ill people are much more likely to take sick leave. In the United States employees with mental health problems are off sick on average for around 11% of the time, compared with 1.5% for the general population. The position is similar in other countries, as table 5.2 shows.[28] Between a third and a half of all days off work are accounted for by mental illness. Sometimes the absence is mainly due to the atmosphere at work, but in at least 80% of cases it is due to an underlying mental health problem that makes it impossible to cope.[29]

And even when people are at work, their mind is not always on the job. In surveys people can be asked how their present productivity compares with the productivity they are normally capable of. From their answers it is estimated that "presenteeism" (that is, substandard performance) accounts for at least as great a loss of output as absenteeism does[30]—and probably more in the case of mental health.

Lower Earnings and Worse Exam Results

For all these reasons and more, it is not surprising that, even when they have work, mentally ill people earn less on average than other people. This emerges strikingly from a study of former recruits to the Swedish army.[31] At the age of eighteen they were assessed for their cognitive ability— their knowledge and their ability to reason. But they were also assessed for their noncognitive skills, in other words for their social and emotional health. These recruits were then followed up in adult life to the age of forty and over, and their earnings were recorded. It turned out that people's noncognitive skills (or lack of them) explained as much of the variation in their earnings as was explained by their cognitive skills. Even when it comes to earnings, heart counts for as much as head.

A similar story applies earlier in life, when we try to explain educational success. In one study, a group of US eighth graders was tested at the beginning of the school year for IQ and for self-discipline. At the end of the year the group members got their school grades. Self-discipline explained twice as much of the variation in grades as IQ did.[32]

Chaotic and Antisocial Behavior

This takes us back to mental health in childhood. How does it affect the rest of our childhood, and how does it predict our subsequent life as an adult?

As table 5.3 shows, children with mental health problems lead very different lives from other children. They are more likely to play truant, more likely to be excluded from school, more likely to smoke or use drugs, and more likely to self-harm. In each case the difference in likelihood is at least four times. And, according to their parents, nearly one in five of these children have physically self-harmed. So we can already see the beginnings of many of our social problems.

Childhood problems frequently lead to similar problems in later life. In table 5.4 we concentrate on children who had behavioral problems when they were really young, aged seven to nine. We take the worst 5% (those with "conduct

Table 5.3. Mental health problems produce other problems in childhood

	Children with:		
	Emotional disorders	Conduct disorders	No disorder
Percentage who			
play truant	16	22	3
have ever been excluded from school	12	34	4
smoke regularly	19	30	5
have ever used hard drugs	6	12	1
have ever self-harmed	19	18	2

(Children 11–16).

Table 5.4. Behavioral problems at age 7–9 predict problems in later life

	Children whose childhood conduct was in	
	Worst 5%	Best 50%
Percentage subsequently		
committing violent offences (21–25)	35	3
drug dependent (21–25)	20	5
teenage parent	20	4
suicide attempt (to age 25)	18	4
welfare dependent (age 25)	33	9

disorder") and the best-behaved 50%, and we then compare their subsequent behavior as adults. The difference is astonishing. The "bad children" were ten times more likely to commit violent crime; four times more likely to become drug dependent or teenage parents, or to have attempted suicide; and three times more likely to be welfare dependent.

This does not mean that all crime or other bad things come from this group of people. (As simple arithmetic shows, the best 50% in the group committed as much violent crime in total as the worst 5%.) But it does mean that, if the worst 5% behaved like the best 50%, we would have very much less crime and welfare dependence, and many fewer drug users, teenage parents, and suicide attempts.[33]

Thus it is not surprising that in the United States a half of all prisoners are already mentally ill when they are sent to prison.[34] In Britain some 50% have depression or anxiety disorders.[35] Some 20% were ill enough to be in treatment for their mental health in the year before they were sent to prison.[36] Mental health problems make it much more likely that you will go to prison. They also make it more likely that, when you come out, you will reoffend within a year.[37]

Mental illness also causes much of the domestic violence that ruins so many families and so many lives. At least a third of those who are violent to their partners are mentally ill.[38] Equally, mentally ill people are much more likely than others to be victims of domestic and other forms of violent crime—in Britain a person with severe mental illness is five times more likely than other people to be a victim of violence.[39]

The Life Course

Thus mental health affects every area of our life. But just how important is it, compared with other things, in determining the most important outcome—how satisfied we are with our lives? To answer this, we shall use a large cohort study that follows children born in 1970 right through their lives.[40]

What affects our life-satisfaction as adults? There are immediate causes and more distant causes, coming from our childhood and earlier life. If we start with the *immediate causes*, the most obvious, apart from mental health, are family income, having a job if you want one, being well educated, being married or cohabiting, not having a criminal record, and reporting good physical health. Figure 5.5 measures how well each factor predicts life-satisfaction (holding the other factors constant). The diagram shows that all the factors matter but that emotional health explains much more of the variation in life-satisfaction than any other factor. As before, we measure emotional health earlier to

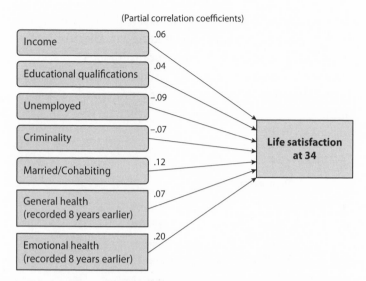

(Partial correlation coefficients)

Income — .06

Educational qualifications — .04

Unemployed — −.09

Criminality — −.07

Married/Cohabiting — .12

General health (recorded 8 years earlier) — .07

Emotional health (recorded 8 years earlier) — .20

Life satisfaction at 34

Figure 5.5. What are the main immediate influences on adult life-satisfaction? These numbers show the strength of the relationship between life-satisfaction and each variable after controlling for the influence of all the other variables shown.

avoid any charge of tautology, and we do the same with self-reported general health.[41]

The next question is about *the more distant causes*—our family background and our development as a child. We focus on three main aspects of people's development as children—their brainpower (test performance), their behavior, and their emotional health. Most broad-minded people realize that brainpower is not everything, but they often think the main other thing is behavior.[42] It certainly matters. But so does how people feel inside—their emotional health.

How much each matters depends on which adult outcome you are looking at, as figure 5.6 shows.[43] A child's test performance is the best predictor of subsequent income and educational qualifications. Behavior is the most important predictor of criminality and finding a partner. And emotional health is the best predictor of health later.

But the ultimate test is what produces a satisfied adult. What best predicts that? It is your emotional health as a child. That is the best predictor of whether you will have

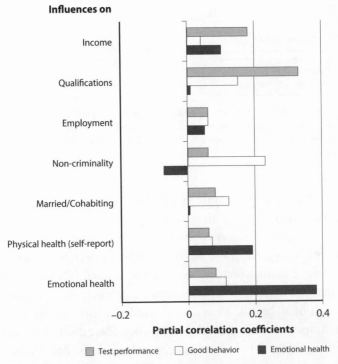

Figure 5.6. What are the main childhood influences on different aspects of adult life?
These numbers show how well each adult variable on the left-hand side is predicted by childhood test performance, good behavior, and emotional health, holding other variables constant.

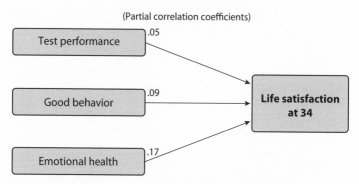

Figure 5.7. What are the main childhood influences on adult life-satisfaction? These numbers show how well life-satisfaction at age 34 is predicted by childhood test performance, good behavior, and emotional health, after controlling for the influence of each other variable. Other variables are female (.07), family economic status (.06), and family psycho-social state (.03).

a satisfying adult life. Next in importance is your behavior. And least important is your brainpower. Figure 5.7 says it all.

These conclusions are strikingly at odds with the priorities of educationists. Of course if their main criterion of a successful life is income, then brainpower should be their overriding concern. But if they care about happiness and misery, they should give much more attention to the emotional health of our children. This is not the same as their behavior—the two are only weakly connected. We are talking about the inner person, whom we too easily neglect. Our mental health is our greatest asset; it is vital for each of us. As Mark Twain once put it, "Of all the things I ever lost, I miss my mind the most."

But our mental health is also vital for the rest of society. Where mental health is lacking, it costs the rest of us a pretty penny.

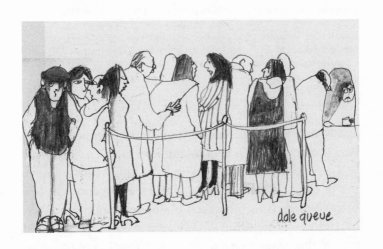

dole queue

6 ∗ The Economic Cost

My daughter is on a yearlong waiting list for treatment.
She's trying to get herself well enough to come off
welfare benefits but the support is not there.

Letter to Richard Layard, March 2012

Mental illness is not just a problem for those it affects directly. It also imposes huge costs on the rest of society. So the case for tackling the problem is not just humanitarian—it is also a matter of plain economics. Mental health problems diminish work, increase crime, and make additional demands on physical health care. What is the cost?

Fewer in Work, and More on Welfare

As we have seen, fewer mentally ill people are able to work. In fact if mentally ill people worked as much as the rest of the population, total employment would be over 4% higher.[1] That would mean billions more in output.

Some of this loss is borne by the individuals themselves, but a substantial amount is borne by everyone as taxpayers. People who do not work pay lower taxes. On top of that many of them get disability benefits; in most rich countries over 2% of the working-age population are on disability benefits because of mental health problems.[2]

There are also many people who do have jobs but have time off sick or who fail to perform to the best of their ability. This involves a major cost for employers. Over 40% of all absenteeism is due to mental illness (and most of this mental illness is unconnected with the atmosphere at work). If mentally ill people were no more absent than other workers, hours worked would rise by over 1%.[3]

There is also "presenteeism," the less effective work done when a person's mind is in a mess. This is more difficult to measure and has been mainly studied by asking people questions about how much below their best they are working. From comparing mentally ill people with others, we can estimate that presenteeism due to mental illness reduces output by at least as much as absenteeism does.[4]

Mental health problems affect the output of the economy through nonemployment, absenteeism, and presenteeism (not to mention the effects on relatives' ability to get out to work). On a conservative analysis, the combined effect is to reduce our national income (GNP) by 4%—almost as much as most countries spend on education. Half of this cost falls on government funds.[5]

More Crime

Much of the crime in advanced countries is done by people with substance dependence and/or a prior diagnosis of conduct disorder. Indeed, a third of all crime is committed by people who already had conduct disorder by the age of seven to nine.[6] What is the cost of crime?

It clearly varies from one country to another. In both the United States and Britain the overall economic cost of crime has been estimated at around 5% of national income.[7] This includes the costs of police, courts, prisons, and protection, plus lost production by prisoners and others. Even if we attribute less than one-half of this to mental illness, it still amounts to some 2% of national income, of which about half is borne by the taxpayer.

It is also interesting to look at the costs on a per person basis. There has been a fascinating follow-up study of children age ten in inner London. By the time he was twenty-eight, a child who had conduct disorder at the age of ten had cost the government $150,000 more than a child without it.[8] And the additional cost to the economy was greater: in one study the cost per child was estimated at $350,000.[9]

More Physical Health Care

Finally, we come to the costs of health care. As we have already seen in chapter 5, mental health problems often make physical health worse—typically increasing mortality by 50% for people with the same initial health conditions. So, not surprisingly, mental health problems also add greatly to the cost of physical health care.

You can see this by looking at the use of physical health care facilities by people with mental health problems and comparing it with other people's usage. Each time, of course, you have to make the comparison for people whose initial physical health situation is the same. When this is done, you find that mentally ill people cost significantly more than others in terms of their physical health care. Figure 6.1 shows some striking figures on depression from the Colorado Access insurance system. The typical finding is that those who have mental health problems use 60% more physical health care services than equally ill people without mental health problems.[10] Again, a figure of 50% or more.

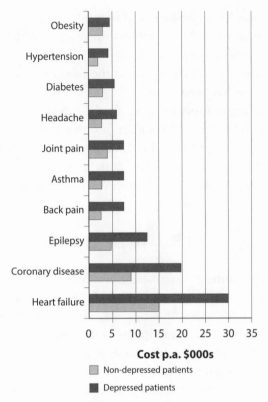

Figure 6.1. Depression increases the cost of physical healthcare.
Costs of anti-depressant prescriptions and mental health treatment are excluded.

This massive extra cost comes about through a variety of channels. For one thing, people with mental health problems do not look after themselves as well—for example, taking less exercise and less regular medication. Their stressed mental state also has direct physiological effects. And finally, mentally ill people are more inclined to worry and there-

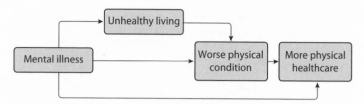

Figure 6.2. Mentally ill people use more physical healthcare than others who start with the same physical problem.

fore to see the doctor. Those three channels are illustrated in figure 6.2.

Besides this there is the related problem of people who have medically unexplained symptoms—they have no diagnosed physical condition but do have serious pain. These people are much more likely to go to the doctor and have more medical tests than the rest of the population. Using a variety of international data, it is possible to calculate the cost of the extra health services used by this group, compared with everyone else in the population.

Not all of these people are mentally ill, and some of their costs are already included in the previous estimate of cost. But even allowing for this, we estimate that the extra physical care of those who are mentally ill costs close to 1% of national income in most advanced countries, and even higher in the United States where health care costs take up so much more of the national income.

In table 6.1 we can begin to put together some estimates of the overall economic cost of mental illness from the three sources we have identified so far. It amounts to some 7% of national income—of which roughly half is borne by the government or by state insurance.

Table 6.1. Economic costs of mental illness

	Cost to the economy	of which, cost to the taxpayers
Non-employment, absenteeism, and presenteeism	4	2
Crime	2	1
Physical health care	1	1
Total	7	4
Mental health care	1	1

(% of national income)

Mental Health Care

To combat these costs, how much do we spend on treating mental illness? The United States spends only 1% of national income and no country spends much more than that.[11] As figure 6.3 shows, most economically advanced countries spend less than 0.5%, and poorer countries very little at all.

For a condition that costs some 7% of national income, we spend only 1% of national income to reduce that cost. On the face of it that does not sound proportionate. But whether it actually is enough depends on whether extra money could be spent effectively. As part two of this book argues, it could.

But where would the extra money come from? For example, if health care budgets are constrained, is there a case for a greater share to go to mental health? As we have seen in rich countries, mental illness accounts for a quarter of the total burden of disease. So what share does it get in health care expenditure? Look at the second chart in figure 6.3.

As % of GDP

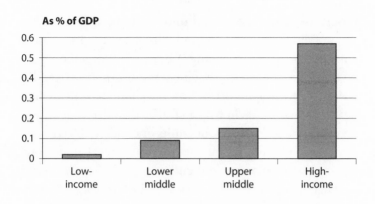

As % of health spending

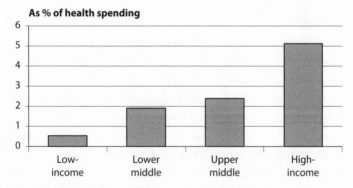

Figure 6.3. Mental health spending is very low in every type of country.

The average rich country spends only 5% of its health care money on mental health. The United States spends around 7%,[12] Britain spends 13%, and most spend a smaller percentage. Since we have cost-effective treatments for mental illness and millions of people who go untreated, this is a clear case of system-level discrimination.

In rich countries the main form of this discrimination is against people with the most common psychological problems—depression and chronic anxiety states. For example, in England more than $150 billion a year goes on total government health spending.[13] But under $6 billion goes on the seven million adults with depression and anxiety disorders,[14] and roughly $1 billion on children with mental health problems. Included in all that is under $1.5 billion on psychological therapy for adults or children. By contrast some $45 billion goes on the physical care of under one million people who are in their last year of life.[15] We spend so much on trying to extend the *length* of life (often by very small amounts), and yet so little on improving its *quality*.

There is also extraordinary discrimination in the allocation of funds for research. In England only 5% of funds for medical research goes on mental health research, and much of that goes on dementia.[16] The situation is similar in the United States.[17] But the biggest scandal is that so few of those in distress are in treatment. Good treatments already exist, but less than a third receive help. Even simple economics says this must change. But first we need to look at how mental health problems come about.

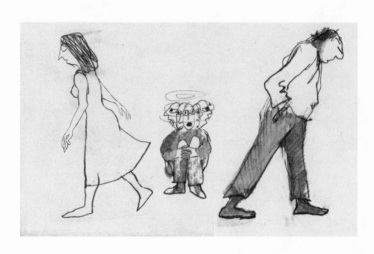

7 * What Causes Mental Illness?

Don't be too hard on parents. You may find yourself in their place.

Ivy Compton-Burnett, Elders and Betters

Like everything else about us, our mental health depends on a mixture of nature and nurture—of genes and experience. All we can change is the experience. But to understand how that works we must also understand the role of our genes.

From Freud the Western world concluded that mental illness was largely because of how our parents behaved. If we resembled our parents, it was because of how they treated us, not the genes they gave us.[1] Until the 1960s that was the received wisdom. But then in 1966 Leonard Heston of the University of Oregon published his classic paper on schizophrenia.[2]

Heston studied people who had been adopted at birth and therefore were brought up by different parents from those who gave them their genes. Some of these adopted people had been born to schizophrenic mothers, while others had been born to "normal" parents. Heston found that, where the biological mother was schizophrenic, 10% of the children became schizophrenic, compared with virtually none of the children of nonschizophrenic mothers.[3] Further work revealed something even more striking. If the biological mother is schizophrenic, it makes no difference whether she brings up her children herself or if someone else does it—either way, 10% of the children become schizophrenic.

These remarkable facts are summarized in table 7.1. They establish beyond question that schizophrenia is partly due

Table 7.1. Schizophrenic mothers have 10 times more schizophrenic offspring, even if they never see them

	% of each group who are schizophrenic
People brought up in adopted family	
With biological mother schizophrenic	10
With biological mother not schizophrenic	1
People brought up by biological mother	
With biological mother schizophrenic	10

to the genes and that the behavior of the parents is not uniquely responsible. If children are like their parents, it is not necessarily because of how their parents treat them.

Since the 1960s it has become increasingly clear that genes play a significant role in all mental illness. They never automatically cause it, but they can substantially affect the risk. We are the product of both our genes and our experience, and of how they interact. So let us look first at the genes and then at the even more important influence of our experience, and at how the two interact.

Our Genes

As every parent knows, children differ from the moment they are born—unless they are identical twins. Yet many people still believe in the "blank slate"—the idea that all that matters is our experience, and what it writes on the slate. In modern times this idea goes back to John Locke, the great English philosopher of the late seventeenth century, who believed that our identity was determined entirely by our experience.[4]

As we have seen, we now know this is wrong. Further evidence against it comes from the study of twins. Some twins are identical—they come from the same fertilized egg and have identical genes. Other twins are not identical and come from two different eggs, fertilized by different sperm. These nonidentical twins have only half their genes in common, while identical twins have exactly the same genes. If genes matter for mental health, identical twins should be more similar in their mental health than nonidentical twins of the same sex.

That is exactly what we find in figure 7.1. If one twin has bipolar disorder, the other twin will also have it in 55% of cases if he is identical, but in only 7% of cases if he is not identical.[5] The reason is quite simply that identical twins have more of their genes in common, and these genes matter.[6]

When it comes to major depression, the role of genes is less, but it is still substantial. As figure 7.1 shows, unipolar

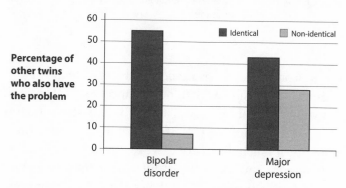

Figure 7.1. If one twin has the problem, does the other have it also? (Same-sex twins.)

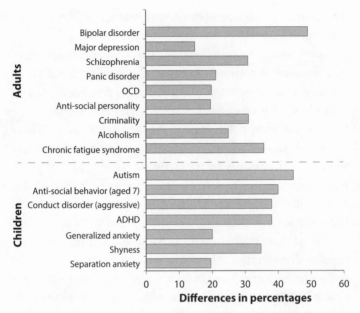

Figure 7.2. Identical twins are more similar than non-identical twins.
For each illness we take same-sex twins who have the illness and ask what percentage of their co-twins also have it. We do this for identical twins and for non-identical twins. This chart shows the difference in the two percentages. For OCD, alcoholism, and all childhood conditions except autism, we give the difference in co-twins' correlations (of continuous measures) rather than co-twins' concordance (of a binary measure).

major depression also has a genetic element—identical twins are much more similar than nonidentical twins. The similarity for identical twins is 43% and for nonidentical twins 28%—a "difference" of 15%. If genes did not matter, there would be no such difference.

In figure 7.2 we show these "differences" for all the main mental health problems. As it shows, they all have some genetic element.

Adoption studies show similar patterns. We have already discussed the evidence on this for schizophrenia. For depression and anxiety, adoption studies yield less striking results, but they are not inconsistent with the evidence from the twin studies we have just looked at.[7]

Genetic evidence is also interesting in helping us identify any common genetic features shared by different conditions. For example, the genes that bring the risk of depression are apparently the same as those that bring a risk of anxiety.[8] It is experience that determines whether the risk is realized and in which form—anxiety or depression. Both of these disorders are "internalizing." By contrast, the risk of "externalizing" disorders, like antisocial disorder or substance abuse, depends on a different set of genes.[9]

How Genes and Experience Interact

Genes matter, but they are only the beginning of the story. They cannot on their own give you a mental health problem. All they do is increase the risk that you will get one. The final outcome depends on experience as well. For example, as figure 7.1 showed, if you have bipolar disorder, your twin with the *same* genes is only 55% likely to be bipolar. That is a high percentage, but it also puts a clear upper limit to the role of genes in explaining who does and who does not become bipolar.[10]

Moreover, that figure only tells us the role of genes under existing social arrangements. If we had better treatments for bipolar disorder or a more mental-health-conscious society, the figure might well be very different. So it is time we turned to the role of experience, which—unlike our genes—is something we can change. (Gene therapy is unlikely to become widespread any time soon.)

One of the basic messages coming from modern science is that genes and experience interact in determining who you become. In other words, there is not simply a part of you that is due to your genes and another part that is due to your experience: bad genes amplify the effect of bad experiences, and vice versa.[11]

This is true in many animals. If young rats are blindfolded at birth and only exposed to light six months later, they never develop proper sight.[12] The genes for sight only work when there is enough light at the right time. Or take the case of phenylketonuria in humans. This is a disease that produces mental retardation, but you only get the disease if you have the gene and you eat phenylalanine (which most of us do—it is a protein present in many common foods). If you have a different diet, you don't get the disease even if you have the gene.

Thus experience is crucial for our development. It not only affects us directly but it also turns our genes on or off. This can be traced at the physical, molecular level through the new science of epigenetics. It can also be observed at the psychological level by seeing how the impact of bad genes interacts with bad experiences.

Clear evidence comes from studies of adopted children. For example, one study looked at antisocial behavior in adolescents. This was more common if the adoptive parents were antisocial, but the effect was greater still when the biological parents were also antisocial.[13] So there is gene-experience interaction. Similar results have been found in many other studies of the mental health of adopted children when they were more grown up.[14]

But the most striking examples come from studies that use each individual's DNA. We are now at a stage where individual genes have been identified that can predispose to depression or bad behavior. One such gene is the serotonin transporter gene, which regulates the flow of serotonin in the brain, which in turn affects the risk of depression.

For this gene, as for all others, people have two codings (or alleles). One coding comes from the father and the other from the mother. For the serotonin transporter gene the codings can be either short or long. Short codings are more likely to produce depression than the longer variant. So the worst situation is when both codings are short and the best when both are long. But the gene only exerts its effect if the person is also exposed to enough bad life events.

This is illustrated in figure 7.3. The more short codings a person has the more likely he/she is to become depressed— but *only* if the experience is also bad enough. Similarly, bad experience only matters if you have bad enough genes.[15]

These results can be reproduced experimentally. When humans are subjected to stress, those with the most short codings show the most activity in the amygdala—the emotional part of the brain.[16] And when macaque monkeys are separated from their mothers, those with the most short codings show the most stressed reactions.[17]

The results reported in figure 7.3 come from a classic study by Avshalom Caspi and Terrie Moffitt of Duke University. They used data on twenty-six-year-olds followed from birth in Dunedin, New Zealand. Caspi and Moffitt also studied what determined antisocial behavior in those same adults. In this case they focused on the gene for monoamine oxidase A (MAOA), which is involved in the metabolism of the chemical neurotransmitters that transmit signals in the brain. People with the low MAOA genotype were more likely to become antisocial adults, but only if they had been maltreated as children (see figure 7.4). Similarly, maltreatment had a much worse effect if you had the "bad" gene.

These studies have had major influence. They have not always been replicated in other data, but the balance of subsequent research confirms their basic message.[18] Although genes and environment have independent effects, they also interact—in the sense that bad genes amplify the effect of bad experiences, and vice versa.

Crucially, the reverse is also often true. If you have bad genes, you also respond better to good experiences.[19] For example, children who have the short codings for serotonin respond better to CBT than other children do.[20] This is immensely encouraging. The fact that genes affect us does not mean we can do nothing to offset their effects. On the

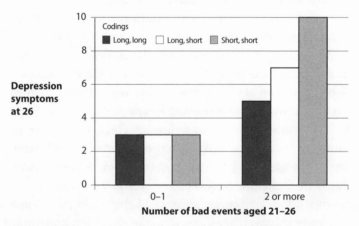

Figure 7.3. Depression: the impact of bad events depends on the serotonin transporter gene.
Past-year depression based on Diagnostic Interview Schedule.

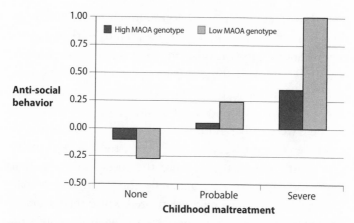

Figure 7.4. Anti-social behavior: the impact of childhood maltreatment depends on the MAOA gene.
Composite index of anti-social behavior (z-scores). Aggregate of four measures: adolescent DSM IV, convictions, violent personality at 26 (self-assessed and assessed by contacts).

contrary, if our genes are against us, we may become *more* responsive to good interventions on our behalf.

Our Personal Experience

What are the main experiences that affect our mental health? With animals in a lab it is extremely easy to pin down the effect of experience, because we can vary it experimentally. For example, we can investigate the effect of parenting by randomly allocating some animals to different parents. A classic study of rats by Michael Meaney took the offspring of mother rats who were bad at licking their offspring and allocated some of them to foster mothers who were good at licking.[21] These offspring grew up to be much less stressed, and they also became much better at licking their own offspring. Similarly, a classic study of rhesus monkeys by Suomi took the offspring of overactive mothers and randomly allocated some of them to calmer foster mothers.[22] These offspring became much calmer than those who stayed with their biological mothers.

These were truly randomized adoption studies. With humans we cannot do such experiments, and when we compare most individuals, we have the messy situation that genes and experience are generally correlated. The people with "bad" genes generally get treated worse than average. They may also themselves choose worse environments. And in any case, when they are born, they had parents who shared some of their genes and who created a home environment that was affected by those genes (unless their children were adopted away).

This makes it more difficult to disentangle the effects of experience. But it remains essential that we do so because that is what we can try to change. And we have many sources of evidence to help us do this from adoption studies to twin studies to studies of the same individuals over their lifetime (when the genes stay put but the environment changes). From all of this some clear lessons emerge. These are that our childhood and family experience matter but they are not all. Our well-being also depends on our adult experiences, our physical health, our work, and the kind of society we live in.

Childhood[23]

The best protection against mental illness is positive parenting—a harmonious relationship with at least one adult who is totally committed, dependable, and appreciative. A child needs to be loved, and to become attached to an adult. If a child is subject to physical abuse, that child is about six times more likely than average to become an abusive parent.

This is an important risk factor. But it does not mean that all abused children become abusers. On the contrary, two-thirds of abused children do not themselves become abusers. This is true of all traumatic experiences: many people emerge relatively unaffected, but for some, life is truly blighted. Those people who report significant emotional abuse in child-hood are three times more likely to become depressed as adults, but even so 40% do not.[24] When bad things happen, some people are just more vulnerable than others.

A second key issue for children is the relationship be-tween the parents. Family discord is bad for the mental health of a child, and parental separation adds to the prob-lem except where the discord was already intense.[25] There is no evidence that parental separation causes less damage now than when it was less common.[26] Mental health prob-lems can also arise if either parent becomes mentally ill, or addicted to alcohol or drugs.[27]

What if the mother works and puts the child in child care? There is no evidence of large negative effects, though some US evidence suggests that long hours of nursery care can make children slightly more aggressive and antisocial.[28] However, the effects are small unless at the same time basic parental love diminishes.

Children can also develop mental illness as a result of their own physical illness and of bullying at school. And what about child poverty? It seems to have no direct effect per se on a child's mental health, once the other factors we have mentioned are taken into account. But it will of course have an influence insofar as it leads to worse parenting or worse mental health for a parent.[29]

So we know a good deal about how family upbringing affects mental illness, and also something about what form the mental illness takes. Depression depends on a sense of helplessness, which can easily become ingrained if a child has no control over what happens.[30] Similarly, anxiety can be provoked by insufficient protection or by overprotection. And bad behavior is undoubtedly encouraged by witnessing it in the parental home. Such problems often continue into adult life. But what are the effects of adult life itself?

Adult Life Events

As we have seen, most anxiety disorders appear by the time of adolescence. But depression mainly begins in adulthood. How far is it caused by events in the person's life? This was first studied carefully by George Brown, who showed that depression often came after a series of bad experiences such as the death of a loved one, domestic violence, separation from a partner, job loss, or an illness in the family.[31] Moreover, ongoing difficulties in life circumstances can also make depression more likely. For example, mothers with three or more young children at home are more likely to become depressed. By the same token, good experiences make depression less likely. For example, a woman who has a close confidante is less likely to become depressed when bad events occur.

Physical Illness

One problem that can cause acute depression or anxiety is physical illness. An acute episode can certainly trigger mental illness, and is one of those bad life events we have already referred to.[32] But a long-term condition like diabetes, heart pain, or breathlessness can also produce ongoing mental illness, and as many as one-third of people with serious long-term physical conditions also have mental problems that need addressing[33]—and often aren't.

Work

As social animals, people need to be needed—by their families and by the community around them. Work can also provide an important source of feeling needed. By contrast, unemployment and job insecurity are well-documented sources of mental illness, and unemployment is a condition to which most people do not adapt as it continues.[34] But work alone is not enough—the environment at work is also important for mental health. We know that some workplaces are hellish to work in. A hostile workplace can easily cause a mental collapse. By contrast, in a healthy workplace people are given clear goals, but also the maximum possible autonomy in how they achieve these goals. At the same time support and appreciative feedback are essential.[35] It makes all the difference if you feel that your colleagues are on your side.

Social Class and Income

What about social class? There is some association between mental illness and social class, but it is much less than is often thought. Table 7.2 gives the basic figures for Britain, using a standard survey of people in their homes. The first column shows what percentage of people with depression

Table 7.2. Mentally ill people are drawn from all social classes

Social class	People with depression or anxiety disorder (% in each class)	People without depression or anxiety disorder (% in each class)
1	3	5
2	27	29
3 Non-manual	25	24
3 Manual	19	19
4	18	16
5	7	5
Total	100	100

and anxiety disorders come from each social class. As you can see, they are drawn from every social class. But so is the rest of the population, as shown in the second column. Among those who are depressed there is a rather higher proportion in the bottom social classes (4 and 5) than there is in the general population. And there is a rather lower proportion in the top social class (class 1). But the problem is very much present in all classes.

Moreover, in looking at the relation between mental illness and social class there is an obvious problem of causality since mental health problems can push you down the occupational ladder. This may be less true of IQ, which is why in table 7.3 we repeat the analysis using IQ. Here again the association with mental illness is quite weak.

If we turn to income, there is little doubt that this does affect a person's physical health. But the effects on mental health are much less clear.[36] In those studies where there is an association, there is the standard issue of whether income is causing mental health or vice versa. However, for children this is not a major issue since we are talking about the parents' income and the mental health of the child. While it is well established that low family income damages the educational performance of children, there is no similar finding about its effects on mental health. For example, the British survey of child mental health showed no effect of income on child mental health once the other variables we have discussed are controlled for. This was so both in comparing individuals at a point in time and also when examining how children's mental health changed when family income changed.[37]

We can also get some evidence on this issue from the effect of interventions aimed at improving mental health. One study compared a set of programs that directly tackle mental illness with another set of programs that attempt to tackle it indirectly by improving incomes. The first set of experiments were markedly more successful—and they also indirectly improved incomes.[38]

Table 7.3. Mentally ill people are drawn from all levels of ability

Level of IQ	People with depression or anxiety disorder (% at each IQ level)	People without depression or anxiety disorder (% at each IQ level)
120 and over	5	8
110–119	21	23
100–109	21	26
90–99	28	25
80–89	18	14
Under 80	7	5
Total	100	100

A Lesson in Statistics

There are many known causes of mental illness, which we have described. If we want to reduce mental illness, should we attack its causes, or simply treat it when it appears? Obviously both. Mental health should be prevented if possible (the public health approach) and treated when it arises (the treatment approach). But how successful are both approaches likely to be?

Advocates of the public health approach are prone to exaggerate its power by using a particular statistical device. For example, consider the world described table 7.4. There are 100 people of whom 20 have a characteristic (like having a depressed mother) that gives them a high risk that they will become mentally ill. In the event 10 of them do become so. But 10 do not. And, in addition, 10 people who were not high risk in fact become mentally ill. How could we describe this situation? Well, the risk of mental illness is 50% for the high-risk group and only 12.5% for the low-risk group. So it is four times higher for the high-risk group. Or if we use the "odds ratio" (which statisticians prefer) the odds are seven times higher for the high-risk group than for the others.[39]

That sounds pretty decisive. Obviously, you might think, the way to deal with the mental health problem is to work on the high-risk group before they become ill. But wait a minute. Even if you were completely successful in preventing mental illness among those at high risk (which is quite unlikely), you would only have halved the number of mentally ill people. And you would have also spent a lot of unnecessary effort on those high-risk people who would never have become ill in the first place.[40]

Table 7.4. Not all high-risk people become mentally ill, and many low-risk people do

	Mental illness?		
	Yes	No	Total
Risk?			
High	10	10	20
Low	10	70	80
Total	20	80	100

Whether the effort is worthwhile depends on the cost, compared with the cost of other desirable objectives. In many cases preventive interventions are worthwhile even if some of the effort was unnecessary. But notice that in our particular example there are no more people who actually become mentally ill than those who are at high risk. Clearly the moral obligation is strongest toward those who actually become ill, which is one reason why we claim that this is the highest priority. And they should be treated quickly. If they become ill as children, they should be treated then. That form of "early intervention" has the top priority, while "early intervention" on high-risk groups who are not yet ill has, we believe, a lower priority.

But is there some additional reason for wanting to know the causes of mental illness? Of course there is. Everyone wants to know why they are the way they are. And, equally important, this can be an important element in treatment.

But at that stage a second issue arises. Many people have experiences that put them in the high-risk group. But, as the table shows, some of them do not emerge as mentally ill. They were surely shaken by their experiences. But, while some who go down stay down, others recover. So a key question is, what makes mental illness persist for some but not for others? We can address this issue by taking a simple example.

What Makes Mental Problems Persist?

In 1998 a splinter group of the Irish Republican Army exploded a bomb in a crowded shopping street in Omagh, Northern Ireland. Many people were traumatized. They had all been through roughly the same experience. Yet only some people had enduring problems. Why was this?

Overwhelmingly, the best predictor of whether a person would continue to suffer was the way they thought about and reacted to the trauma.[41] As figure 7.5 indicates, those with negative thoughts and behavior continued to suffer while those, initially the same, whose thinking was more positive were much more likely to recover. The same is true of other forms of anxiety or depression—those who recover are those who are least preoccupied with themselves.

This provides important clues to treatment. It is not always necessary to know the originating cause of a problem in order to help someone. But it is essential to know what is maintaining the problem. As it happens, the same distinction often applies in physical medicine. It may not be necessary to know what caused the cancer—you cure it by cutting it out. And it may not be necessary to know why this person has blocked arteries—you cure the breathlessness by putting in a stent. Indeed, people have run marathons with a stent—the originating cause has not been tackled but

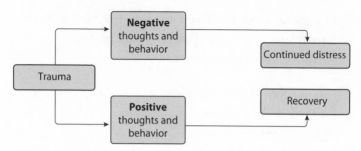

Figure 7.5. Why some recover and others do not.

the immediate problem has. Similarly, infections are often cured with antibiotics, without knowing their causes.

The Nature of Society

We have talked so far as if mental illness was a purely personal phenomenon. But it is also of course affected by the ethos and culture of a society. To understand how this works, we have to compare countries, and we can do this using the Gallup World Poll.[42] It asks people in every country the following question about their level of mental distress.

> [on mental distress] Did you experience the following feelings a lot of the day yesterday? (Yes/No): Worry, Sadness, Anger, Depression

We can assign for each country a mental distress measure based on adding together the responses to the four emotions.

The survey then asks the following questions about people's experience of their community, and counts the proportion of respondents saying yes:

[on social support] If you were in trouble, do you have relatives or friends you can count on to help you whenever you need them, or not?

[on freedom] In your country, are you satisfied or dissatisfied with your freedom to choose what you do with your life?

To measure the prevalence of corruption, they count the average proportion of respondents saying yes to the following two questions:

Is corruption widespread within businesses located in your country, or not?

Is corruption widespread throughout the government in your country, or not?

According to the poll, countries differ greatly in their degree of mental distress. As we have seen in chapter 3, there is no relationship between this and the level of national income per head.[43] But there is a clear and significant relationship between the level of mental distress and the answers to the questions about social support, freedom, and corruption.[44] Other studies have also found good relationships between national well-being and trust.[45] In fact people at all income levels benefit greatly from a civilized and caring community. So Maslow's famous phrase is not right—there is not a "hierarchy of needs," where satisfying higher needs makes no difference until lower needs are satisfied. The ethos of a country matters greatly for mental health at all levels of income.

But what about the specific issue of income inequality? Comparing a limited number of countries, Oliver James, author of *Affluenza*, has found a strong correlation between income inequality and mental illness.[46] But, before drawing any conclusion, one has to include a range of other variables, and in careful work with many variables John Helliwell of the University of British Columbia has failed to find any clear impact of income inequality on any measure of national well-being or negative emotion (other things constant).[47] It is certainly important to live in a society where people trust each other. But an ethos of mutual respect and equal value is probably more important than the precise distribution of income.

Health Inequalities

Within any country there are of course sharp inequalities in physical health between different income groups—another argument for reducing income inequality.[48] But these inequalities are not the only inequalities in the world of health. Perhaps the most extreme inequality is between people who are mentally ill and people who are physically ill. Most physically ill people get treated, and most mentally ill people do not. This is a very specific problem and it could be dealt with in less than ten years. It is surely the top priority in health care.

Most of those affected are suffering from depression or anxiety disorders, or from conduct disorder in childhood. So that is our central focus for the rest of this book.

We know a great deal about how to treat these problems and we also know what kinds of social change would produce a less distressed society. We should use both types of knowledge. We need changes at both levels—individual and social. The social changes are discussed in chapters 15 and 16. They will take time. Meanwhile the most urgent task of all is to treat the untreated mental illness already staring us in the face. That is the subject of the next six chapters.

PART TWO

What Can Be Done?

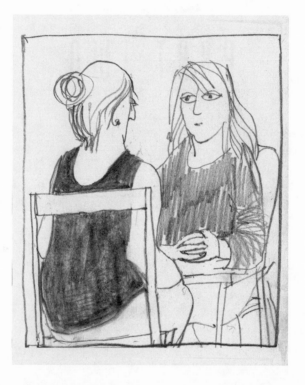

8 * Does Therapy Work?

Canst thou not minister to a mind diseased,
Pluck from the memory a rooted sorrow,
Raze out the written troubles of the brain.

Macbeth, *Act V, Scene iii*

Until the 1950s there were no scientifically validated treatments for most mental health problems. But then came striking drug discoveries, and in the following decades major advances in psychological therapy. These advances were made by using the same standard methods of scientific experiment that are used in treating physical illnesses. As a result we now have a range of treatments for mental health problems that have high success rates—as high as the success rates in treating many physical problems.

To ensure that people get the best treatments, most countries have bodies that issue clinical guidelines. One of the most widely respected internationally is England's NICE— the National Institute for Health and Care Excellence. Its job is to review the scientific evidence about the different treatments available for every problem, physical as well as mental. It assembles widely representative panels of experts from all clinical professions and the public. The National Health Service is meant to provide the treatments they recommend.

So how do they judge which treatments are the most effective? And which treatments do they recommend?

The Scientific Approach

To tell whether a treatment works, it is not enough to see that many people get better—they might have gotten better anyway. Instead we have to compare the people who were treated with people who were not treated. For example, it might seem likely that after a gruesome traffic accident the injured people would benefit from an immediate debriefing—an opportunity to go over in detail what happened in the accident and how they feel about it. And indeed many of those debriefed feel better in the days that follow, and think the debriefing helped them. But when a proper comparison is made with people who have not been debriefed, it turns out that people fare better on average if they are not debriefed. The reason is that debriefing refocuses attention on the traumatic incident, which for many people is counter-productive. Figure 8.1 shows the findings of a study on highly traumatized road traffic accident victims taken to a local hospital.[1] Most improved, but those who had been debriefed improved less.

Some people recover naturally—the mind heals itself. So if your patients recover, it does not mean that you have helped them—even if they think you have. They may have recovered naturally. Of course every professional treasures successful outcomes, but to be certain that you have made a difference there has to be a process of comparison. It is easy for therapists to believe they are helping when they are not. For two thousand years, doctors took liters of blood from infected patients and believed they were helping them. But in fact they were making them worse—George Washington may have died as a result.[2] There are countless examples of interventions that seemed plausible but that, after proper

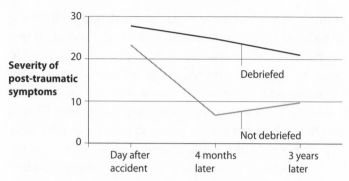

Figure 8.1. Debriefing after a road accident can increase PTSD.
Persons with high stress levels after the accident. Severity is measured by the Impact of Event scale, the Brief Symptom Inventory, and an authors' questionnaire.

comparisons, were found to have done no good or even harm.[3]

The gold standard for comparison is the randomized controlled trial, or RCT. In this case a single collection of patients (or clients, if you prefer) is split randomly into two groups. One group is given the treatment and the other, the control group, is asked to wait for treatment ("wait list"), *or* given a placebo, *or* given "treatment as usual." We then compare the outcomes for the treatment group and the control group. Ideally the experiment is double blind: the people measuring the outcomes do not know who was and was not treated, and the people treated do not know whether they were treated specially. Not all RCTs can be double blind, but even if they are not, they are preferable to any other form of experiment.[4]

If the two groups are selected in some other way, we can of course allow for the ways in which we know they differ. But it is never possible to allow for differences that cannot be measured and yet could be affecting the outcomes. For example, when hormone replacement therapy (HRT) was introduced for postmenopausal women, it was noticed that people who took it were less likely to develop heart trouble. But these were a self-selected group, and to find out whether HRT was actually reducing cardiovascular disorder it was necessary to allocate people randomly between HRT and no-HRT. When this was done, it was found that HRT actually increased cardiovascular disorders rather than reducing them.[5] Proper trials are crucial to finding out what difference treatments really make.

Until the 1950s no proper trials were done on methods of treating mental illness, and few pre-1950 treatments have been shown to have any effect.[6] But since the 1950s, powerful new methods of treatment have emerged—both drugs and psychological treatments.

Pills

In 1952 it was found that an antihistamine called chlorpromazine helps people with schizophrenia, and a range of further discoveries have made it possible for most people with this condition to lead more tolerable lives, usually outside the hospital. Also in the 1950s lithium was found to help people with bipolar disorder, and together with subsequent discoveries, it has helped millions to experience fewer extreme periods of mania or depression. These new drugs for psychotic patients are one of the major ways in which modern science has been able to reduce unbearable human pain.

But, as we have said, this book is mainly about the much larger number of people suffering from unipolar depression and anxiety disorders. The first effective antidepressant was a tricyclic drug called imipramine. This was discovered in the 1950s, and though subsequent second-generation anti-depressants have succeeded in reducing side effects, they have produced little improvement in the rates of recovery through treatment. The main use of antidepressants is for moderate to severe depression, where the proportion who respond well after four months on medication is some 50%, compared with around 30% of people who took a placebo tablet.[7]

However, a major problem with depression is the danger of subsequent relapse. It turned out that the relapse rate after recovering with antidepressants is about the same as (or worse than) after spontaneous recovery. So there is no evidence of any enduring effect. But the relapse rate can be reduced by continuing to take antidepressants. NICE recommends that all patients with severe depression should be offered antidepressants during their depression and for a period thereafter. But NICE does not recommend anti-depressants for mild or moderate depression, since there is no evidence that on average they make a difference. For these more mild depressions only psychological treatments are recommended. It is deeply worrying that about 8% of adults in Europe are now taking antidepressants,[8] since most people who take them have only mild or moderate depression.

For patients with anxiety disorders, the first major drug was Valium, one of the benzodiazepine class of tranquilizers (which also include most sleeping tablets). Valium was not intended as a treatment, but rather as a system of on-going support—"mother's little friend." The problem was that it was addictive. Nowadays the main drug treatments for anxiety disorders are antidepressants. These are recommended by NICE. But with anxiety disorders psychological treatments are generally more effective, particularly in terms of long-term relapse prevention.

All psychological therapies have the same ultimate aim—to help the patient to help herself, to empower her, and make her able to control her own life. Of all the therapies, cognitive behavioral therapy (or CBT) is the most developed in terms of the evidence of its effectiveness. It is not the only evidence-based therapy, and many more therapies will emerge in the future. But at present CBT is the only therapy that is recommended by NICE for both depression and all types of anxiety disorder. We shall begin by focusing on it before we discuss the full range of evidence-based therapies in later chapters.

Cognitive Behavioral Therapy

The first key assumption in CBT is that our thoughts affect our feelings. This was what Aaron Beck observed in his depressed patients in Philadelphia. They were constantly ruminating with "automatic thoughts" going round and round in their head.[9] These thoughts were often biased in a negative direction and reflected the core beliefs people had about themselves and the world. These beliefs were causing the depression or anxiety disorder. By getting people to articulate their automatic thoughts, Beck was able to get people to examine and question their core beliefs. And frequently they got better.

He called his treatment cognitive therapy because it centered on people's thoughts (or cognition) and how these affect their feelings. It is also of course true that feelings affect thoughts. But in Beck's experience the best way into this vicious circle was by trying to change the thoughts.

In saying this, Beck is in line with much of the wisdom of the ages. As the Stoics pointed out, what disturbs us is not what happens to us but how we react to it.[10] Buddha said much the same thing. The aim is to achieve control over your thoughts, and in this way to achieve control over your life. So what is new about cognitive therapy? Two things.

The first is the *systematic structure* of the treatment. It is not only a series of ideas but also a structured practice focused directly on the core problem experienced by each person. First comes the cooperative relationship (or therapeutic alliance) between therapist and patient, without which nothing can happen. Then in the sessions (usually no more than fourteen to twenty) issues are raised in a well-tested sequence, with homework assignments between sessions. The whole treatment is based on manuals, which provide a range of options to the therapist. The therapist's practice is also subject to regular supervision.

The second characteristic of CBT is the *use of measurement and the experimental method* to find out exactly which approaches work best. Beck himself developed one of the first and best-known scales for measuring depression, the Beck Depression Inventory. He then organized one of the first randomized trials of psychological therapy for depression, which showed that CBT did better than imipramine both at the end of treatment and a year later.[11] In many subsequent trials CBT has been found to do at least as well as antidepressants—with roughly 50% recovery rates—but, as figure 8.2 shows, CBT leads to much longer periods free of relapse.[12] So the charge that CBT is just a sticking-plaster is

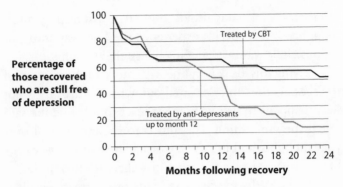

Figure 8.2. CBT reduces the recurrence of depression better than anti-depressants do.
In this experiment one group of depressed patients were given CBT and another anti-depressants. After treatment ended, patients who had recovered were followed for 24 months. Patients originally treated with anti-depressants continued this treatment for 12 months after recovery.

simply wide of the mark. Those who benefit regain lasting control over their lives and their emotions, which is what they wanted.

In fact *brain research* reveals something very interesting about how CBT works.[13] Most depressed people differ from other people in two ways. First, their amygdala is over-reactive (this is the structure deep in the brain that, for example, promotes the fight-or-flight response). Second, much of their prefrontal cortex is underactive (this is the "more conscious" region that normally regulates our emotions and reactions). However, it turns out that after depressed people have had CBT, their amygdala becomes less over-reactive. This is shown in figure 8.3. The top line shows how depressed patients respond when bad things are suggested about them. The next line down shows how the same patients respond after treatment. They become much the same as the normal controls in the third line. The analysis also shows an equally powerful effect of CBT in increasing activity in the prefrontal cortex.

Interestingly, antidepressants have the same effect on the amygdala, but much less on the prefrontal cortex. This may explain why antidepressants work well while they are being taken—they directly affect the amygdala, which is the "seat of the emotions." But once you stop taking them, they have no effect. By contrast, CBT has an ongoing effect even after treatment, because it has helped to reestablish the control of the prefrontal cortex over the amygdala. The neuroscience here is in its infancy but the results are suggestive.

Depression is not of course the only common mental illness. Anxiety conditions are equally common, and for them modern psychology had been developing a very different approach—using more behavioral techniques. Even before Beck's work, Joseph Wolpe and colleagues had found that phobias could frequently be cured by gradually increasing exposure to the feared situation. It was natural in the

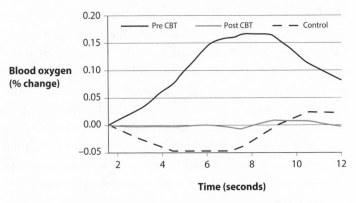

Figure 8.3. After CBT the brain's blood oxygen response to negative words becomes normal.

decades that followed that the cognitive and behavioral strands came together. Treatments for depression incorporated more purely behavioral elements—in "behavioral activation" depressed patients are asked to do three things a day, such as take some exercise, talk to someone, and do something they like. And treatments for anxiety incorporate more cognitive elements—becoming aware of "safety behaviors," and questioning what might happen if the safety behavior was not followed.

At the same time other therapies were being developed and subjected to similar standards of testing: interpersonal therapy, couples therapy, brief psychodynamic therapy, and, of course, counseling. Where the evidence is in their favor, these too are recommended by NICE. In the next chapter we discuss CBT in more detail, and in chapter 10 we discuss the full range of other therapies.

Effectiveness in the Field

But first there are three general issues that apply to all therapies. The first is whether treatments developed in a clinical research environment can really be transplanted into the field—and implemented successfully week after week and year after year. It is sometimes said that clinical trials are done on atypical populations of patients, and that they are done by better therapists than could be found more generally. However, there have been many studies of clinical practice in the field, and they show similar levels of outcome to those in clinical trials—provided the treatment is the same.[14]

In fact the issue of exclusion criteria has been greatly exaggerated. It is true that clinical trials often use exclusion criteria to focus very specifically on the problem to be dealt with. But one key trial of CBT for obsessive-compulsive disorder (OCD) took patients who had been excluded from previous trials on various grounds. When these patients were treated, the results were as good as in the previous trials on the more restricted range of patients.[15]

It is of course a worry if therapists are not properly trained. But they can be trained in large numbers, and in chapter 12 we show how England's Improving Access to Psychological Therapies program has achieved results approaching those in clinical trials.

Do the Effects of Therapy Last?

The second issue is whether the effects of therapy last. All psychological therapies aim to help people learn to cope with difficult events and emotions. Does such learning help people stay well in the future? Long-term follow-up studies are difficult to conduct, so they are less common than studies of the immediate effects of therapy. However, there is good evidence for enduring benefit.

In anxiety disorders follow-up studies of one to nine years have shown that although people's anxiety can fluctuate, on average people who were treated with CBT are as well at follow-up as they were at the end of therapy.[16] For around one in five people this sustained benefit may have been facilitated by having some booster treatment. In social anxiety disorder, some studies have even shown further improvement during follow-up,[17] perhaps as a consequence of people's reduced levels of anxiety enabling them to make new friends who further boost their confidence.

Depression is a recurring problem, with many people who have had one episode being at risk for a future episode. Two psychological therapies (CBT and behavioral activation) have been shown to halve that risk, compared to treatment with antidepressants.[18] For people who were treated with medications initially, completing a course of mindfulness-based cognitive therapy after they recover also approximately halves their risk of a future relapse.[19]

The Therapy or the Therapist?

Another issue is how much it matters which therapy is used. Many people allege that it is not the therapy that matters but the therapist: "A good therapist will achieve results whatever therapy they practice, provided they believe in it." They also produce evidence that they believe supports this argument. For example, there have been audits of routine clinical services that found that there is little relationship between the type of therapy a clinician says they delivered and the outcomes their clients achieve.[20]

However, this type of evidence is seriously flawed. First, in such audits therapists only submit data on a fraction of the patients they see—the data may be quite unrepresentative. Moreover, there is generally a systematic upward bias in the measurement of outcomes, because most of the therapists have not been using session-by-session monitoring. We know about this bias from the experience of the program of Improving Access to Psychological Therapies described in chapter 12. In its first year the program collected not only session-by-session data on depression and anxiety (assessed by PHQ-9 and GAD-7) but also more detailed (CORE-OM) data from questionnaires administered before and after treatment. However, many of the patients did not complete the second, posttreatment questionnaire. It turned out that the patients who did complete that questionnaire had double the improvement (on PHQ-9 and GAD-7) of those who did not.[21] This is striking evidence of the upward bias that partial response can cause. For this reason routine studies end up exaggerating what is achieved.

A second problem with these audits is that different therapists may see different types of patients, since there is no randomization between therapists. And third, there is no guarantee that therapies were appropriately delivered— a recent audit of routine delivery of psychological therapies in England found that for some non-CBT therapies 30% or more of therapists said they were not trained to deliver the treatment they were providing.[22]

When therapists vary in their level of training, their results vary enormously. But when all the therapists have been equally well trained in the therapy they are delivering, there are quite small differences in the results they achieve.[23] Personality differences play a surprisingly small role.

So the same therapist can perform much better if trained in an effective therapy. Here is an example. A group of counselors treating panic disorder were achieving only 22% recovery.[24] They asked for training in CBT and were given an intensive three-day course followed by eight months of supervised practice. After this, as figure 8.4 shows, they were achieving 68% recovery rates, close to those in standard clinical trials.

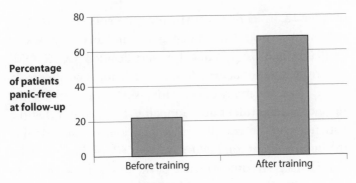

Figure 8.4. Training therapists in CBT can improve recovery rates.

So the therapist's character is less crucial than you might think. But what about the therapy? Some people claim that it does not matter which therapy you practice, provided you believe in it.[25] But one imaginative experiment directly addressed this issue. In Germany the preferred treatment for social phobia has been cognitive therapy at Frankfurt, but at Freiburg it has been interpersonal therapy. So therapists

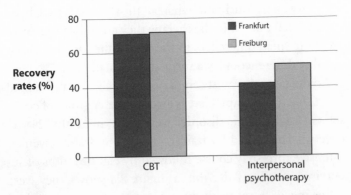

Figure 8.5. For social phobia, CBT does better than interpersonal psychotherapy, whichever group of therapists provide it.

in both centers agreed to a four-part experiment in which each group of therapists would use each therapy (on different groups of patients).[26] The result was clear cut and is shown in figure 8.5: CBT did better than interpersonal therapy at both centers. Even therapists who worked at the center that focuses on interpersonal therapy got better results with CBT. So the same people, with the same empathy, got different results when they practiced the different therapies. This shows that the therapy does matter.

How are therapies developed and how do they work? In the next chapter we focus on CBT, and in the one after on the full range of evidence-based therapies.

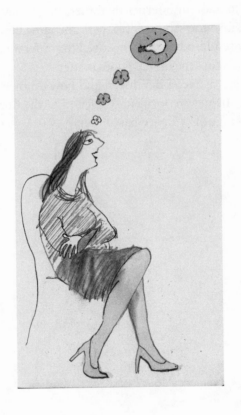

9 * How Therapies Are Developed

> Men are disturbed not by things, but by the view they take of them.
>
> *Epictetus*

In the beginning was Freud. He was the founder of talking therapies—and in particular of listening therapies. He, more than anyone, taught therapists to listen. His writings about the unconscious caught people's imagination and stimulated a wonderful flourishing of new ideas in literature and art during the early twentieth century. The concept of the "talking cure" was born.

However, psychoanalysis—the therapy that Freud advocated—has not been shown to be effective. Freud thought the main cause of many mental health problems was the repressed memory of traumatic events in early childhood. To cure them, people needed to gain insight into the links between the repressed memories and their current feelings. A lengthy course of therapy, often extended over several years, was considered essential for recovery.

Many people say they have benefited from this treatment. But it lasts so long that the natural recovery rate for the conditions being treated is also high, and there are no randomized controlled trials that have shown that psychoanalysis does better than natural recovery.[1] Moreover, the length of the treatment makes it so costly that it could never be provided to most of those who need help. For these reasons, Freud's followers have developed and evaluated briefer forms of "psychodynamic" treatment, which are recommended by NICE.

The Behavioral Revolution

In fact it was not until the late 1950s that the first therapy emerged that science showed to be effective. This was systematic desensitization, developed by the South African doctor Joseph Wolpe. Like Freud, Wolpe thought that phobias (and many other mental health problems) might have their origins in traumatic events. However, he did not think that people had to gain insight into the origins of their problems if they were to recover. Instead, he emphasized the way in which our current patterns of behavior might maintain the problem, and he therefore focused on changing the maintaining behavior.

Wolpe was much influenced by Pavlov's earlier studies of learning in animals. In a classic experiment, Pavlov had given dogs a mild electric shock to the paw, which made them flinch. He then, shortly before the shock, presented the dogs with various "neutral" stimuli, like the ringing of a bell or the shining of a light. After a few pairings of the neutral stimulus with the shock, the dogs had an emotional response (of freezing) whenever the previously neutral stimulus was presented. Pavlov used the term "conditioning" to describe the process by which the neutral stimulus was converted to one that evoked an emotional response. He also experimented with ways of abolishing the acquired emotional response and found that, if the sound or light was repeatedly presented without being followed by a shock, the emotional response was lost.

Wolpe hypothesized that people with phobias might have developed their excessive fears of particular objects (heights, small animals, strangers, and such) through conditioning, and hence could be treated by repeatedly exposing them to the phobic objects without the trauma occurring.[2] He was concerned that this behavioral treatment might be excessively stressful, so he developed a modified extinction procedure in which people were taught to relax and then exposed in imagination to the fear-evoking stimuli. When the fear of the imagined object declined, people were encouraged to expose themselves to the real thing.

In the 1960s Gordon L. Paul of the University of Illinois conducted the first ever randomized controlled trial of a psychological therapy to find out whether systematic desensitization worked.[3] He randomized people with a phobia of public speaking to five weeks of either systematic desensitization, or insight-oriented therapy based on Freud's ideas, or no treatment. The people who received systematic desensitization improved considerably more than those who received insight-oriented therapy or no therapy at all. Many subsequent trials confirmed the effectiveness of Wolpe's treatment for phobias, and the idea that emotional problems might be overcome by changing one's behavior in line with the principles of conditioning theory were successfully applied to a range of other anxiety problems, including obsessive-compulsive disorder. In the process, it was discovered that Wolpe had been excessively cautious in his approach to therapy. It proved unnecessary to train patients to relax before exposing them to the feared situations. And it was generally found that exposure in real life, rather than imagination, was the most effective procedure.

Beck and Cognitive Therapy

Following their early successes with some anxiety disorders, the behaviorists turned their attention to depression. Patients were encouraged to systematically engage in potentially pleasurable activities. But this approach was not particularly successful. Thankfully, Aaron Beck was working on an alternative strategy, which was much more promising. As we have seen, Beck had originally trained as a psychoanalyst but was frustrated by the slowness of that method of therapy. He had studied the content of dreams among depressed patients, hoping to identify some of the unconscious conflicts specified by Freud. However, he found that the content of depressed people's dreams was remarkably similar to the themes behind many of their daytime thoughts. In particular, he noticed that the thinking of people who were depressed could be characterized as a triad comprising a negative view of themselves ("I am a failure"), of their world ("People don't care about me"), and their future ("Bad things always happen to me"). In contrast to prevailing psychiatric wisdom, he suggested that such negative thoughts were not simply a symptom of depression. Instead, they were crucially involved in maintaining the condition.

This idea led him to develop a distinctive form of treatment called "cognitive therapy," in which the therapist helps the patient to question their negative thoughts and to replace them with more realistic thoughts, when appropriate.[4] While a fair amount of cognitive therapy for depression could be described as a "talking therapy," Beck also emphasized the importance of changing behavior in order to help people change their beliefs. For example, someone who persistently believed that they were a failure would be encouraged to reengage with activities they had been avoiding in a graded way, so they could start to reexperience success and regain confidence.

In 1977, Beck and colleagues published the first randomized controlled trial of cognitive therapy for depression.[5] The results stunned the psychiatric world. Cognitive therapy was significantly more effective than treatment with the leading antidepressant. Many subsequent trials have clarified the comparison of cognitive therapy with medication. Overall, these indicate that cognitive therapy and antidepressants are similarly effective in the short term. But, as discussed in the previous chapter, patients who are treated with cognitive therapy are less likely to relapse.[6] As depression is a recurring condition, the reduction in relapse is crucial. During cognitive therapy, people learn skills for managing their negative moods, which reduce the chance of their becoming depressed when things next go wrong in their lives. By contrast, antidepressants do not reduce your risk of a future episode of depression, once you have stopped taking them.

Cognitive Behavioral Therapy

The success of Beck's combination of cognitive and behavioral therapy had an enormous impact. Since the 1980s dozens of researchers have been inspired by his work and have developed theoretical models of different mental health conditions that highlight the way in which distorted thinking and changes in behavior combine to maintain the problem. Therapy then focuses on changing both thinking and behavior, and hence it is usually called cognitive behavioral therapy.[7]

Much of the success of cognitive behavioral therapy results from its firm foundation in basic psychological research. In each of the conditions to which it has been applied, researchers asked the question: "What keeps the problem going?" The psychological processes they identify when answering this question then become the main targets for the therapy. This is in marked contrast to Freud's view that successful treatment should focus on identifying the origins of a mental health problem. The way in which research on "maintaining factors" has led to better treatments is well illustrated by the case of panic disorder, particularly since it used to be considered one of the least treatable psychiatric conditions.

Panic Disorder

A panic attack is a sudden surge of anxiety that often only lasts a few minutes but can be quite devastating. Individuals experience feelings of breathlessness, a racing heart, dizziness, and many other sensations. Typically, they think they are in danger of dying, having a heart attack, fainting, losing control, or going mad. Many people have had occasional panic attacks. But if you have panic disorder, you experience repeated attacks and you become extremely fearful of further attacks and the harm they might do you. Many people experience their first panic attack in crowds or on public transport, and therefore they tend to avoid these situations— some become completely housebound. One-fifth of people who have panic attacks attempt to kill themselves.[8]

The novelist Shiva Naipaul experienced his first panic attack while an undergraduate. In his autobiography he vividly describes the experience.

Strolling along Saint Giles, I was neither happy nor sad. I may have been thinking how pleasant it would be to get hold of a punt, to spend an hour or two on the river. Approaching Broad Street, I suddenly became aware that something peculiar was happening to me. Inexplicably, my heart had started to race, my palms to moisten with sweat, my head to swim. I realized I was terribly afraid. But afraid of what? What was there to be so afraid of on this soft, blue afternoon? Dazed, barely able to maintain my balance, barely able to breathe, I huddled against the wall of Balliol. The summer sky, so benign, so unthreatening, was transformed into a wheeling amphitheatre of undefined menace; a maelstrom of annihilating vacuity. Staring at it, wave upon wave of raw fear swept through me. I imagined myself a body: a nameless corpse to be picked up from the street. It was as if all the secret terrors accumulated from birth had broken loose of their chains and come upon me in one overwhelming, retributive flood. How long I remained huddled against that wall, I cannot say. Maybe no more than a minute or two. The worst of the panic receded. In its place came exhaustion, a sensation of such utter weariness and debilitation that, for an interval, I could do nothing at all, lacking even the small amount of strength required to lift my arms and dry my sweat-soaked forehead.[9]

Naipaul's account nicely highlights the unexpected nature of his panic attack. It seemed to come out of the blue. This feature initially led psychiatrists to think that panic disorder is a result of some form of biological abnormality and to advocate drug treatment. However, a simple psychological account was soon developed, and it has proved highly successful.

In the psychological account[10]—the "cognitive model of panic disorder"—it is proposed that individuals who experience repeated panic attacks do so because they tend to misinterpret normal bodily sensations, thinking that something serious is about to happen to their body ("I am having a heart attack") or to their mind ("I am going mad"). This misinterpretation makes them more afraid, and their body reacts to the fear by generating more sensations (racing heart, dizziness, and so on), which make the person even more convinced that something terrible is about to happen. Figure 9.1 illustrates the process.

Actually, nothing bad does happen. People do not die or go mad in a panic attack, and the symptoms usually subside after a few minutes. Yet many people with panic disorder experience repeated panic attacks, which raises the question: why don't people learn that their panic attacks are harmless? The cognitive model has an answer to this question. It suggests that when people are afraid, they do things to try and prevent what they are afraid of from happening. These are "safety behaviors." The terrible thing wouldn't have happened anyway, but since it doesn't the patient is confirmed in the belief that it was the safety-seeking behavior that prevented it. The fears continue.

So, for example, a patient who feels dizzy in a supermarket and fears that she will collapse may hold her cart firmly until the dizziness subsides and believe that this is the reason why she did not collapse. She will therefore be similarly afraid next time she feels dizzy. However, if she had moved away from the cart and stood unsupported, she would have

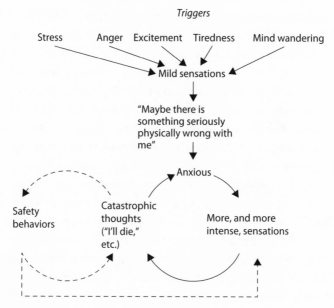

Figure 9.1. How fear builds up in panic attacks.

discovered that the dizzy feeling would not lead to her collapsing and is harmless.

People who suffer from panic attacks often notice small changes in their body (missed heartbeats, tingling, and such) and tend to think this means there is something seriously wrong with them. They often seek extra physical investigations and reassurance from their family doctor. The cognitive model also has an explanation for the perception of the small changes. Because of their fears, people with panic tend to focus their attention on their bodies and, as a consequence, become very good at spotting slight changes that other people would not have been aware of.

An elegant experiment by the German psychologist Anke Ehlers nicely illustrates this point.[11] She asked some people to sit quietly in a room and count their heartbeats without taking their pulse. Everyone found the task difficult and made mistakes. However, people with panic disorder made significantly fewer mistakes. In other words, their fears made them more attentive to their bodies, which made them better than the rest of us at following their heartbeats. Unfortunately, this enhanced attention came at a price. Over the following year those who were particularly good at spotting their heartbeats continued to suffer from panic attacks, while those who made more errors tended to recover.[12]

The cognitive model of panic, and the research studies that tested it, generated a distinctive form of cognitive behavioral therapy that has proved highly effective and is now recommended by NICE as a leading treatment for the condition.[13] Therapy starts by reviewing a recent panic attack and deriving a personal version of the model with your own thoughts, sensations, and safety-seeking behavior.

John, a man of thirty-two, had been having panic attacks on most days for the last three years. His main fear was that the chest pain, palpitations, and shortness of breath he experienced in his attacks meant he was having a heart attack. His safety-seeking behaviors included sitting down and resting during an attack ("to take the strain off my heart"), taking acetaminophen (which he falsely believed would stop a heart attack), and focusing his attention on his heart. He had also changed his lifestyle since developing panic disorder. He used to exercise regularly but had now stopped. Also he would only have sex with his partner in the mornings, when he felt rested. Both of these changes in lifestyle were driven by his belief that he had to protect his heart.

With the help of his therapist, John devised a model of his problem that is shown in figure 9.2. Therapy focused

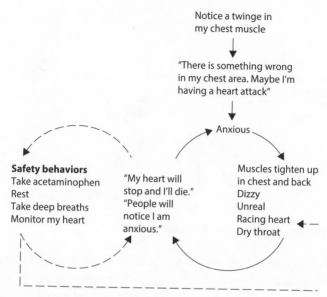

Figure 9.2. John's model of his panic attacks.

on helping John understand that the problem was not his heart but a mistaken belief, which generated anxiety and bodily sensations in a vicious circle. In discussion with his therapist he noticed several things that were a better fit with the vicious circle idea. He noticed that if something very distracting happened during a panic attack (such as a winning goal from his favorite soccer team), all the sensations went away. He agreed this is very unlikely to happen in a real heart attack. He also noticed that dwelling on his fearful thoughts often triggered the attacks, and he agreed that thinking on its own was unlikely to cause a heart attack.

With his therapist, he also planned a series of exercises to help demonstrate to himself that his fears were unrealistic. He jogged along the street outside the clinic with his

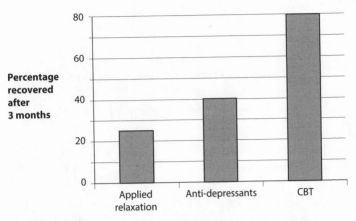

Figure 9.3. For panic disorder CBT gives the best results.

therapist, and they sprinted together with his heart racing. Nothing bad happened. This gave him the courage to return to regular exercise (cycling and soccer with friends), which made him feel even better. He and his partner also returned to having sex when they both wanted to, rather than when John felt most relaxed. Together, these cognitive and behavioral interventions completely stopped John's panic attacks, and after a year he was still fine.

The improvements that John experienced are very much in line with the statistical results of cognitive behavioral therapy in randomized controlled trials for panic disorder. In one trial CBT was compared to a simple psychological coping technique ("applied relaxation") and optimal medication (an antidepressant).[14] Although the applied relaxation technique and the antidepressant both made a difference, many fewer people recovered (25% and 40%) than with cognitive therapy (80%). Figure 9.3 highlights the difference. Furthermore, as with depression, these benefits were maintained well after the end of therapy. While 40% of people who recovered on medication relapsed over the next year, only 5% of those who received cognitive therapy relapsed. The difference in relapse rates was due to the difference in what people had learned. In particular, the people who got cognitive therapy were less likely to interpret bodily sensations as signs of a serious physical problem, and this is what explains their better results.

Brands of CBT

Cognitive behavioral therapy is often discussed as though it is a single therapy. Nothing could be further from the truth. There are in fact many cognitive behavioral therapies, each a highly specialized intervention for a particular problem. They all share a focus on relieving mental suffering by helping people reexamine their most distressing thoughts and change their behavior. But the processes involved in maintaining different emotional problems are subtly different and so therefore are the most effective therapies.

This point can be illustrated by comparing the treatment of panic disorder with the treatment of social anxiety disorder, which is the most common of all the anxiety disorders. In panic disorder the main focus of people's fears is on physical disaster, something bad happening to one's body. In social anxiety disorder, people's fears focus on social disaster.

Social Anxiety Disorder

Social anxiety disorder affects at least 4% of people in any one year and up to 12% of people during their lifetime.[15]

In one study 22% of people with social anxiety were found to have attempted suicide.[16] Many of us are shy in certain situations, but social anxiety disorder goes well beyond that. Situations that people with social anxiety disorder find difficult include meeting strangers; talking in meetings or in groups; starting conversations; talking to authority figures; public speaking; and working, eating, or drinking while being observed. They persistently worry that they will do or say something they will find humiliating or embarrassing. For example, that they will look anxious, blush, sweat, or sound boring or stupid.

Social anxiety disorder can interfere with most areas of life. Educational achievement can be undermined;[17] earnings are reduced;[18] sufferers are less likely to marry or have children;[19] they have more medical outpatient visits;[20] take more days off work;[21] and can have difficulty with everyday activities such as visiting shops, buying clothes, having a haircut, or using a mobile phone while being overheard.

Many people with social anxiety report having been teased or bullied at school. However, as adults they often get positive feedback from other people. Despite this, their fears persist. Why? Three factors may be particularly important.[22]

The first relates to attention. Normally when we meet other people, our attention focuses on them. The opposite happens in people with social anxiety disorder. They become more focused on themselves, trying to imagine how they appear to the other person. The result is disastrous; even if the conversation goes well, the individual with social anxiety disorder may not notice this or benefit from the positive experience. Figure 9.4 shows how people with social phobia focus on themselves when faced with the challenge of speaking to an audience in a few minutes' time.

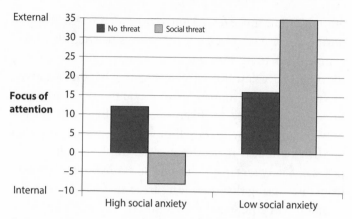

Figure 9.4. Under social threat, anxious people focus on themselves.

Second, while focusing on themselves, people become aware of internal information (anxious feelings and images), which they mistakenly take as good evidence for their worst fears. One of the most common fears is that people will see that you are anxious. People with social anxiety disorder look much less anxious than they feel, but they tend to believe that their feelings are a good indicator of how they look. Images also play a prominent role. When particularly anxious, people with social anxiety disorder report seeing themselves in their mind's eye as though from an observer's perspective. Unfortunately, what they see is not what the observer actually sees but instead is a visualization of their worst fears. So someone who is concerned about blushing may have turned a mild pink in reality, but in their mind's eye, will see themselves as beet red with large white globules of sweat dripping from their forehead.

A third mechanism is the use of safety-seeking behaviors. As in panic disorder, these are motivated by a desire to prevent or minimize feared outcomes (such as "I will appear boring"). For example, someone who is worried that other people think them stupid may try to remember everything the others have said and compare it with what they are about to say to ensure it sounds "clever enough." If the conversation goes well, they are likely to think afterward that was only because of the extra self-monitoring they performed. So their basic fear that other people think they are stupid persists. Safety-seeking behaviors like this prevent people from discovering that their fears are excessive. They can also "contaminate" the social interaction by making it appear as though the person with social anxiety is not interested in, or dislikes, other people. This in turn will elicit less friendly behavior from others.

So how is social anxiety treated? NICE recommends a very specific approach.[23] The therapy starts by helping patients discover that their current strategies for managing social anxiety are not helpful. A role-play in the therapy session shows them that focusing attention on oneself and engaging in safety behaviors makes one feel more anxious. Video feedback helps people to discover that their images of themselves are excessively negative. Training in externally focused attention helps people reduce their self-awareness and become more involved in conversations. Together with their therapist, patients plan experiments in which they can test out their beliefs in action.

For some people, these techniques are supplemented by therapeutic work dealing with early socially traumatic experiences. The negative images that people experience often have their roots in these events, and therapy may focus on helping people break the link between the past trauma and their current experience. For example, someone who was

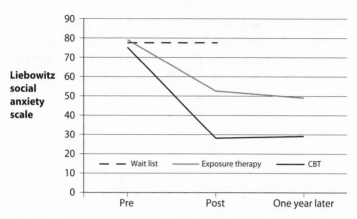

Figure 9.5. Social anxiety responds to CBT better than to exposure therapy.

frequently criticized in front of other children by hypercritical adults may have difficulty dealing with authority figures at work. Once this cause is established, a simple technique might involve selectively focusing on everything about the authority figure at work that is different from the critic in one's childhood. If this is not helpful, more detailed discussion of the early trauma may be indicated in order to reduce its emotional impact.

As we saw at the beginning of this chapter, Gordon Paul's seminal randomized controlled trial of Wolpe's systematic desensitization focused on social anxiety disorder and showed that exposure-based treatment was effective. More recent cognitive models and the research that underpins them have further increased the possibility of effective treatment. As we can see from figure 9.5, the latest forms of cognitive therapy achieve substantially better outcomes than the exposure-based treatments originally developed by the behaviorists. Some 78% of patients recovered with cognitive therapy, compared to 38% with exposure therapy.[24]

Other randomized controlled trials have established that cognitive therapy is superior to antidepressant medication and several other equally plausible alternative psychological treatments, such as interpersonal psychotherapy and psychodynamic psychotherapy.[25]

Conclusion

Therapies differ. But they also have much in common. These include raising hope, providing a secure, confidential environment to discuss one's problems with a friendly person, and developing a practical plan. These features, which were clearly articulated by the psychologist Carl Rogers, probably explain why most therapies are better than nothing at all. However, for many conditions the things that distinguish one therapy from another are also important. They must explain why some therapies work better than others in achieving the same objective.

The main differences are in the mechanisms the therapies assume. For example, in panic disorder CBT assumes that the main mechanisms are negative thoughts and safety-seeking behaviors. It is these that the therapy aims to change. But can we show empirically that CBT actually changes those mechanisms, and that that is how it succeeds when it does?

To answer this question requires mediation analysis, which is still in its infancy in psychological therapy research. However, early findings are generally consistent with the theoretical models on which the treatments are based. For example, in the randomized controlled trial of panic disorder shown earlier, the greater reduction in panic achieved by cognitive therapy compared to medication and relaxation training could be explained by the former's greater impact on patients' negative beliefs and safety-seeking behaviors. Similarly, in the randomized controlled trial of social anxiety disorder, the greater reduction in social anxiety disorder achieved by cognitive therapy compared to exposure therapy could be explained by the former's greater impact on negative beliefs, self-focused attention, and safety-seeking behaviors.[26]

Enough on CBT. We have focused on it so far because it is the most widely researched form of psychological therapy. But there are many others, and some have proved equally effective for some conditions, especially depression. These therapies provide patients with a range of choices, and as time goes by, will no doubt become increasingly important as more research leads to ever better ways of treating psychological problems.

What is the full range of evidence-based therapies that are now recommended?

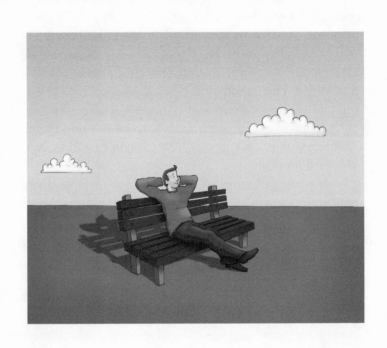

10 * What Works for Whom?

It often feels as if I have been reborn

Gareth[1]

In looking at what works, we take NICE to be our guide. Many professional organizations (such as the American Psychiatric and Psychological Associations, and the Institute of Medicine) have produced treatment guidelines and they are generally similar in their recommendations. However, NICE is particularly respected for its approach to evaluating clinical evidence. For each disorder they have a committee drawn from clinicians and researchers of all persuasions, as well as service users, who agree on what treatments should be recommended. First, the committee's statisticians summarize the evidence using standard techniques, mainly meta-analyses. They give priority to the results of randomized controlled trials but also use other forms of supporting evidence. On the basis of the evidence, the committee then agrees on their recommended treatments. The three tables in this chapter show what they recommend for adults with mental health problems.[2] We begin with depression, anxiety, and eating disorders.

Depression

As we have seen, depression is one of the most common mental health problems. In it people have a pervasive low mood and also often lack energy, have difficulty concentrating, lose interest in things, have disturbed sleep,

Table 10.1. NICE's recommendations for the psychological treatment of depression, anxiety, and eating disorders

Condition	Treatment
Depression: moderate to severe	CBT or Interpersonal psychotherapy, each with anti-depressants
Depression: mild to moderate	CBT (individual or group)
	Interpersonal psychotherapy
	Behavioral activation
	Behavioral couples therapy
	Counseling for depression
	Short-term psychodynamic therapy
Panic disorder	CBT
Social anxiety disorder	CBT
	Short-term psychodynamic therapy
Generalized anxiety disorder	CBT
Obsessive-compulsive disorder	CBT
Posttraumatic stress disorder	CBT, EMDR*
Bulimia	CBT
	Interpersonal psychotherapy
Anorexia	In-patient weight-gain program
	CBT
	Interpersonal psychotherapy
	Cognitive analytic therapy

*EMDR = eye-movement desensitization reprocessing therapy (considered by many to be a form of CBT).

are critical of themselves, and feel hopeless about their future. There can be a serious risk of suicide.

A first episode of depression is often triggered by an adverse life event (loss of a job, break-up of a relationship, death of a loved one) or by chronic stress (ongoing financial difficulties, bullying at work). The episode may last just a few weeks or it may last many months. With time the vast majority of people will recover, even without treatment. However, 60% of people who recover will have at least one further episode of depression at some stage in their lives, and for some there will be multiple episodes or they will develop a chronic depressed state.[3] As the number of episodes a person experiences increases, it becomes more and more likely that another episode will come "out of the blue" with no triggering event. So the purpose of treatment is both to speed recovery *and* to reduce the chance of another episode.

Speeding Recovery

Depressive episodes vary in severity. For the treatment of all levels of severity NICE strongly recommends one of two psychological treatments—cognitive behavior therapy or interpersonal psychotherapy. In severe depression it is suggested that these psychological treatments are combined with antidepressants. In mild to moderate depression they are recommended as sole treatments, and medication is not recommended.

Cognitive behavioral therapy for depression focuses on two of the main things that contribute to the maintenance of the depression—negative thinking and the way we behave. With the help of a therapist, people learn how to spot and challenge unhelpful patterns of thinking (such as "I'm a failure," "Things are hopeless"). They also learn to identify and change avoidance behaviors. Because they lack energy and feel nervous or hopeless, depressed people tend to withdraw from many of the activities that previously gave them a sense of pleasure and meaning. But this means that little can happen to help lift their mood. They may also put off dealing with pressing problems. So in therapy, people are encouraged to become more active ("behavioral activation") and are also helped to break problems down into manageable chunks. Treatment mainly focuses on the present but can also address painful memories when these are contributing to the problem. Therapy is very practical, works toward clearly specified goals, and includes "homework" assignments that people do between therapy sessions. For mild to moderate depression, group CBT is also recommended as an option, but there have (surprisingly) been no trials of group therapy compared to individual therapy.

Interpersonal psychotherapy for depression was developed by a New Haven–Boston psychotherapy group led by Myrna Weissman and Gerald Klerman. It is based on the idea that depression often arises from difficulties in relationships with other people. The depression can also affect those relationships. As in cognitive behavioral therapy, treatment starts by providing people with information about depression, its symptoms, how common it is, and its natural course. Therapy then moves on to look at the range of relationships (work, leisure, romantic, home life) that people are involved in, and helps them understand how their mood is linked to their contacts with other people. Several different types of current relationship difficulty might be identified: conflict with another person, life changes that affect how you feel about yourself and others, grief and loss, difficulty in starting or keeping relationships going. Together with a therapist, people identify new ways of dealing with their relationship difficulties and try these out in action.

For mild to moderate, but not for severe, depression, four other psychological therapies are also recommended by NICE. They are behavioral activation, behavioral couples therapy, counseling, and short-term psychodynamic therapy.

Behavioral activation has many similarities to cognitive behavior therapy but more closely focuses on helping people change unhelpful behaviors and become more active.

Behavioral couples therapy for depression is recommended as a possible treatment if the depressed person has a partner and the relationship is felt to be contributing to the depression. Both parties must want to work together in the therapy. Its main focus is on helping the couple understand the effects they have on each other, especially when one partner is depressed. The couple is encouraged to experiment with changing how they communicate and behave toward each other, so that the relationship can become more supportive and mutually fulfilling.

Counseling has a long tradition in psychotherapy and encompasses a range of approaches. The evidence shows that the most effective counseling involves a nondirective approach in which the therapist mainly focuses on current problems and provides a warm and supporting relationship within which people can explore how they feel and think about a number of issues. As advocated by Carl Rogers and others, the therapist generally resists telling people what to do in a particular situation but aims to help them make sense of their experiences and explore new ways of looking at themselves and at the world around them.

Short-term psychodynamic therapy draws on psychodynamic theories developed by Freud and others but is also influenced by other briefer and more structured forms of therapy. It is similar to other therapies in the sense that it aims to help people deal with troublesome feelings and thoughts that are distressing them. However, it places a greater emphasis on helping people see how their present difficulties may be related to previous relationships or other difficulties, and it assumes that previous attempts to avoid painful topics mean that people may not be fully aware of what is distressing them. Short-term psychodynamic psychotherapy is less directive than cognitive behavioral therapy. People are encouraged to explore their feelings about current and past events and to become more aware of what may be the underlying cause of their distress. Therapists may comment on apparent links between present and past events to help people spot recurring themes and self-defeating behaviors, which people may then be motivated to change. It is assumed that some conflicts that have occurred in a person's life will also be mirrored in their relationship with their therapist, which can then be used as a vehicle for change. Therapists try to be as neutral as possible, giving little information about themselves. This is intended to increase the chance that important relationships from the person's past or present will be reflected in their relationship with the therapist. There is much less emphasis on learning particular skills for coping with emotions (keeping thought records, problem solving, and such) than in cognitive behavioral therapy.

Reducing the Risk of Further Depressions

Two psychological treatments that have been shown to reduce the risk of a further episode of depression are recommended by NICE for this purpose. They are cognitive behavioral therapy and mindfulness-based cognitive therapy.

As we have seen, people whose acute episode of depression was treated with cognitive behavioral therapy are 50% less likely to have a new episode in the next two years than people who are treated with antidepressants. Steve Hollon, a psychologist at Vanderbilt University, has shown that cognitive behavioral therapy's superior long-term effects are due to its ability to teach people different ways of thinking about themselves and the meaning of adverse life events.[4] In particular, cognitive behavioral therapy is more effective than medication in reducing depressed people's tendency to see life's setbacks as their fault and a reflection of their personality. It is possible that some of the other psychological treatments that are recommended for acute depression may have similar long-term benefits, but this has not yet been established.

CBT is sometimes given as a prophylactic to patients who have just recovered from depression through the use of antidepressants. The results can be striking and very long lasting, as figure 10.1 shows.[5]

Mindfulness-based cognitive therapy is another exciting new development that can be used to reduce the risk of relapse in people whose depression is treated with medication. It is recommended for people who have had three or more previous episodes of depression. By attending a course of group mindfulness-based cognitive therapy while you are not depressed you can develop skills for dealing with emotional difficulties that approximately halve the likelihood of a new episode of depression. People learn to become more aware of the bodily sensations, thoughts, and feelings that are associated with downward shifts in mood. They learn healthier ways of responding by accepting, but becoming

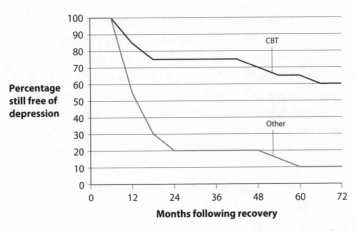

Figure 10.1. Patients who recover from depression are less likely to relapse if given CBT.

less emotionally involved in, those thoughts and feelings. For example, they learn that "thoughts are not facts" and that you can accept difficulties without being overwhelmed by them. Daily practice in mindfulness-based meditation is strongly encouraged.[6]

Anxiety

Cognitive behavioral therapies are effective in all anxiety disorders and are strongly recommended by NICE. For most anxiety conditions, the best cognitive behavioral therapies have been shown to be superior to other psychological therapies that involve as much therapist contact and are as plausible.[7] We can therefore be confident that some of the benefit is due to the specific procedures in each cognitive behavioral therapy, rather than more general features of therapy such as having a warm, supportive and encouraging therapist. In all of the anxiety disorders, CBT helps people to identify what they are afraid of and to test out their negative beliefs in active ways, as we saw in the last chapter. Behavioral experiments are a prominent part of the treatment. Despite these common elements, the most effective CBTs are quite specialized, with certain techniques being used in one anxiety disorder but not in another.

Panic disorder is characterized by repeated, unexpected panic attacks and a persistent fear of future attacks. We outlined the cognitive behavioral approach to treatment in the previous chapter. Randomized controlled trials have established that CBT is effective in the short term, with 60–80% of individuals becoming panic free.[8] The gains that have been made in treatment are generally well maintained when people are followed up a year or so later. As with depression, people are considerably less likely to relapse following treatment with cognitive behavior therapy than following treatment with medication.[9] The superior sustained benefits of psychological therapy are related to the more profound changes in thinking that it achieves. In particular, psychological therapy removes people's tendency to interpret harmless bodily sensations as signs of serious physical illness.[10]

Social anxiety disorder involves a marked fear of social interaction or performance situations, such as public speaking. Individuals fear that, when they are anxious, they will do or say something that leads to their humiliation or embarrassment. We described a cognitive behavioral approach to the treatment of this condition in the last chapter. Until recently, it was common for people with social anxiety disorder to receive CBT in groups. While group treatment has some advantages in terms of discovering that there are many other people with a similar problem, and in providing opportunities to practice social interaction, the latest research suggests that individual CBT is more effective. As a consequence, individual CBT receives NICE's strongest recommendation.[11] Controlled trials have shown that it is superior to a wide range of alternative psychological therapies (including interpersonal psychotherapy, exposure therapy, and psychodynamic psychotherapy).[12] Around 60–80% of people recover, and therapeutic gains appear to be well maintained after up to five years of follow-up.[13] Although less effective than CBT, there is some evidence that short-term psychodynamic psychotherapy can also be beneficial.[14] For this reason, NICE recommends it as a treatment to consider for people who have failed to respond to CBT and do not wish to take medication.

Specific phobias involve a marked fear of a specific object or situation (for example, heights, flying, animals, receiving an injection, seeing blood). In these cases the core element of CBT treatment involves repeated exposure to the feared situations, during which individuals identify and test out their fearful beliefs. In the case of blood-injury phobia, the best results are obtained with "applied tension," in which exposure to the sight of blood or injury is combined with training in a coping technique that prevents the drop in blood pressure that is unique to this particular phobia.[15]

Obsessive-compulsive disorder involves distressing thoughts or images that people feel compelled to try to "put right" or neutralize. Some people are concerned that the objects they touch may be contaminated and they repeatedly clean or wash themselves. Some people are concerned that they may have failed to do something (turn off the gas or electricity) or may have accidentally caused harm (run someone over) and repeatedly check to see that this has not happened. Others may experience thoughts ("the devil") that they feel they need to neutralize with other thoughts (like thinking about God). A core component of the CBT approach involves encouraging people to come into contact with the things that trigger their distressing intrusions (for example, touching a "contaminated" door handle) while not doing anything to "put things right." With practice, this leads to a marked reduction in distress, especially when combined with other ways of reexamining one's fearful thoughts.

Generalized anxiety disorder is characterized by excessive worry. People find themselves worrying about many things (finance, relationships, work, health, and so on) and feel their worry is out of control. Cognitive behavioral therapies focus on helping people to bring their worry under control and prevent it from intruding into their life. A variety of techniques are used. Problematic beliefs that promote worry ("if I worry about it, it won't happen") are identified and addressed, and fears that underlie worry are discussed. People may be given techniques to restrict worry to particular times of day.

NICE does not recommend counseling for generalized anxiety disorder, but it is sometimes offered. A recent audit of routine practice found that recovery rates are higher for people who receive CBT than for those who get counseling, reinforcing the importance of therapists following treatment guidelines.[16]

Posttraumatic stress disorder is a common result of highly traumatic events such as traffic accidents, physical or sexual assaults, witnessing horrible events, or earthquakes. People find themselves haunted by memories of the traumatic events, go out of their way to avoid reminders, and have heightened levels of arousal. Sleep disturbance is common. For many people, these symptoms decline without any treatment in the first few months after the traumatic event. However, some people do not recover. The best predictors of whether a person recovers are their memories, beliefs, and behavior, and these can be changed.[17] Trauma-focused cognitive behavioral therapy targets these processes and is highly effective, with around 70% of people recovering. They are still recovered a year or so later.

Several effective versions of CBT for PTSD have been developed by researchers in the United States (Edna Foa and Patricia Resick) and the United Kingdom (Anke Ehlers and David Clark). The therapies primarily aim to help people process their memories of the traumatic events, so that they generate less emotion and are less intrusive. This is can be achieved by writing a narrative account of the trauma or by reliving certain aspects of the trauma in imagination while in a safe environment. Therapy also focuses on unhelpful beliefs that people may have developed about themselves ("it was all my fault") or their symptoms ("not being able to control my memories means I am going mad"). People often put their lives on hold following a trauma. Therapy also helps people to "reclaim their lives" by reengaging with things that give them a sense of meaning and purpose.

As we have seen, it used to be common for people to be offered psychological debriefing a day or two after a traumatic event. But research studies have shown that this very early intervention is unhelpful as it slows down natural recovery.[18] NICE therefore does not recommend debriefing. Instead, watchful waiting is advocated, with people only being offered formal treatment if symptoms still persist two to three months after the trauma.

Eating Disorders

Eating disorders can ruin people's lives. They involve a severe disturbance in patterns of eating that undermine health and quality of life. People with bulimia alternate between eating excessive amounts (bingeing) and strenuous efforts to rid themselves of the food (by vomiting, purging with laxatives, or excessive exercise). The way they think about their own worth is excessively dependent on their perception of their body shape and weight. People with anorexia severely restrict their eating and have excessively low weight, which can be life threatening. They have a marked fear of putting on weight and tend to see their body, or parts of it, as being fatter than it is.

For *bulimia*, NICE recommends a specialized form of cognitive behavioral therapy as the first-choice treatment.[19] In randomized controlled trials it has been shown to be superior to several equally plausible psychological treatments, and so it must have a specific effect.[20] Around 50% of individuals fully recover and many others show worthwhile gains, which are largely maintained at follow-ups after a year or so. The treatment focuses on helping people to establish more regular patterns of eating and to change their dysfunctional beliefs about food, weight, body image, and self-worth. For people who fail to respond to cognitive behavior therapy for bulimia or want an alternative treatment, interpersonal psychotherapy is recommended, but clients are told that it takes rather longer (eight to twelve months) to achieve results comparable with those obtained by cognitive behavioral therapy.[21]

There is currently less clarity about the optimal psychological treatment for *anorexia*. When individuals' weight becomes dangerously low, they need to go into hospital to get help with putting on weight. NICE also recommends a range of psychological therapies to be given either on their own or in conjunction with an inpatient weight-gain program. However, the overall outcomes that can currently be achieved in anorexia are not as strong as those obtained with bulimia.

Combining Therapy and Medication

For depression, for many anxiety disorders, and for bulimia, there is good evidence that medication (mainly antidepressants) can help. What happens if psychological therapies and medication are combined? Do they work together to produce even greater benefit? Or do they interfere with each other? The answer is complex.

In moderate to severe depression, combining cognitive behavioral therapy and antidepressants appears to increase recovery rates, and the relapse-reducing effect of cognitive behavior therapy is not undermined. However, in some anxiety disorders the good long-term benefits of psychological treatment can be undermined by the simultaneous taking of medication. David Barlow of Boston University followed up people who have been successfully treated for panic disorder for two years after the end of treatment.[22] Those who recovered with cognitive behavior therapy had a significantly lower relapse rate than those who recovered with antidepressant medication. Unfortunately, those who had combined CBT and medication did no better than those who only had medication, unless the tablet was a placebo. It seems that the active chemical ingredients in the antidepressant in some way interfered with the long-term stability of clinical improvements. Also in bulimia, combined treatment does not appear to be better than cognitive behavioral therapy on its own.[23]

New Ways of Delivering Therapy

Traditionally, psychological therapies for depression and anxiety involve weekly sessions of around an hour, with a course of treatment extended over several months. This can be a considerable time commitment; it may be difficult to fit in with work, and it means that recovery will also take several months. More recently, researchers have been investigating other ways of delivering therapy that may speed recovery and/or reduce the number of times an individual has to attend therapy sessions.

One exciting development is the seven-day cognitive behavioral treatment for posttraumatic stress disorder developed by Anke Ehlers and colleagues in the United Kingdom. Normally, CBT for posttraumatic stress disorder involves up to fourteen weekly sessions over three to four months. Ehlers found that the treatment can be just as effective when delivered over a single week.[24] As a consequence, recovery can be achieved in much less time than with the traditional way of delivering therapy.

Another important development is the scientific improvement of methods of self-study. During psychological therapy people learn a lot about how to deal with emotions, thoughts, and behaviors. But in most areas of life much of our learning is obtained from reading, rather than from talking. With this in mind, self-study-assisted versions of several

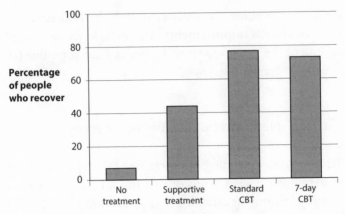

Figure 10.2. For PTSD, CBT delivered in only 7 days is as effective as standard CBT.

cognitive behavioral treatments have been developed. People are given self-study materials to read between therapy sessions. In both panic disorder and social anxiety disorder, the use of self-study modules can double the amount of improvement people make with each hour of therapy.[25] In consequence, fewer visits to a therapist are required.

Low-Intensity Therapy and Stepped Care

If the number of therapy sessions needed for recovery can be drastically reduced by reading self-study materials, it seems likely that some people may be able to benefit from an almost completely self-study-based treatment. In recent years numerous randomized controlled trials have demonstrated that this is the case. Self-help versions of cognitive behavior therapy in which most of the content of treatment is delivered through a book or a computer program have been shown to give significant benefits in mild to moderate depression, in bulimia, and in many, but not all, anxiety disorders.[26] A proportion of people appear to benefit from pure self-help but, in most conditions, higher success rates are achieved with guided self-help. Typically, a health professional provides brief, but regular, support, which may be via telephone, e-mail, and/or text messages, rather than face-to-face sessions.

Thus guided self-help is the obvious first step for mild to moderate depression, bulimia, and some anxiety disorders (but not social anxiety or PTSD). For these people NICE recommends a system of "stepped care" where they are first offered the low-intensity treatments shown in table 10.2 and are only stepped up to the high-intensity treatments in table 10.1 if they fail to respond after several weeks.

Table 10.2. NICE's recommendations for low-intensity psychological treatments of depression, anxiety, and eating disorders

Condition	Treatment
Depression	Guided self-help based on CBT; structured physical activity
Panic disorder	Guided self-help based on CBT
Social phobia	Guided self-help based on CBT is not recommended as a first-line treatment. Consider it only if the person declines face-to-face CBT but is still interested in trying a psychological therapy
Generalized anxiety disorder	Self-help based on CBT; psycho-educational groups
Obsessive-compulsive disorder	Guided self-help based on CBT
Posttraumatic stress disorder	No recommended low-intensity treatment—only watchful waiting
Bulimia	Self-help based on CBT

This approach has proved a good way to maximize the number of people who can be successfully treated in a therapy service with limited resources.[27] However, it is important that it is used properly. In particular, it should not be offered to people with conditions in which low-intensity interventions have not been shown to be effective. And services need to be well organized so that people who fail to recover at low intensity are promptly stepped up to high-intensity therapy. If this does not happen, the overall performance of a service will be poor.[28]

Having discussed the treatment of depression, anxiety, and eating disorders, we now turn our attention to three other disabling mental health conditions: schizophrenia, personality disorders, and alcoholism and drug addiction.

Schizophrenia

Schizophrenia is a relatively rare condition affecting 0.5 to 1% of the population. But it can have a devastating effect on people's lives. People with the diagnosis experience a range of symptoms, and there is debate about whether it is a unitary condition or whether it would be better to talk about schizophrenias. Symptoms are traditionally divided into positive symptoms (such as hallucinations and delusional beliefs) and negative symptoms (such as apathy, disorganized thought patterns, low mood). Most people with schizophrenia are offered antipsychotic medication, which can help reduce the symptoms. However, many people find the side effects of the medication difficult to tolerate and don't consistently take their medication—often leading to relapse. But trials have shown that cognitive behavioral therapies spe-

Table 10.3. NICE's recommendations for psychological treatment of other conditions

Condition	Treatment
Schizophrenia	CBT
	Family therapy
Personality Disorder	
Borderline	Schema-focused cognitive therapy*
	Mentalization*
	Dialectical behavior therapy*
Anti-social	Group-based CBT
Alcohol Dependence	Motivational interviewing
	Behavioral couples therapy
	CBT
Drug Dependence	Motivational interviewing
	Contingency management
	Behavioral couples therapy
	Evidence-based psychological therapy for other problems

*Shown to be superior to standard care or other intervention in at least one randomized controlled trial but not yet specifically recommended by NICE.

cifically developed for schizophrenia can produce beneficial effects on both positive and negative symptoms during an acute episode.[29]

Outside an acute episode, many people with schizophrenia can be helped to lead relatively normal lives. But there is always the issue of relapse. George Brown, a British psychologist, discovered that the family environment in which a person lives has a big influence on whether a person relapses in the face of stress. Individuals who live with people who frequently make critical comments or are highly emotional (technically termed high "expressed emotion" or high EE) are more likely to relapse than people who live in a less critical or emotional household ("low EE").[30] In a landmark study, Julian Leff and colleagues showed that it was possible to teach families who are high EE to become low EE, and this reduces the likelihood that the person with schizophrenia will relapse.[31] Family therapy built on this work has been consistently shown to reduce both EE and relapse.

Psychological treatment has smaller effects on schizophrenia than it does on depression or anxiety. But the gains are still very worthwhile, and it is for this reason that NICE recommends that everyone with schizophrenia should be offered an evidence-based psychological treatment. In the meantime, research on psychological treatments for schizophrenia is very active, and further advances can be expected. A particularly promising approach focuses on individual symptoms (such as hallucinations or delusions) and on the psychological mechanisms that underlie them.

Personality Disorders

The term "personality disorder" is controversial. Sometimes it is used in a pejorative sense, which is quite wrong. When used properly, it refers to long-standing, consistent ways of thinking and behaving that date back to childhood and cause substantial distress to ourselves and other people. Two personality disorders—borderline and antisocial—have attracted most attention in terms of psychological treatment research, and some helpful approaches are now available.

Borderline personality disorder is characterized by unstable relationships, moods, and feelings about oneself, along with a strong tendency to impulsive behavior, some of which is self-destructive (cutting oneself). Currently, NICE does not recommend a particular psychological treatment, as not enough randomized controlled trials have been published to single out a particular approach. However, it is clear that any effective treatment needs to be fairly long term (one year or more) and involves building a strong supportive relationship with the individual and acting in a way that does not risk enhancing his/her fear of being abandoned by others. There are three treatments that have been shown to be effective in a small number of controlled trials, and it seems likely that, as more trials accumulate, they will become more strongly recommended. *Schema-focused cognitive therapy*, based on the work of Jeffrey Young and colleagues in New York, uses many of the techniques of cognitive behavior therapy with an additional focus on reparenting and dealing with early memories of trauma. In one trial schema-focused therapy was compared with an equally plausible psychodynamic treatment.[32] Both were delivered over a period of three years. Forty-six percent of people recovered with schema-focused cognitive therapy, compared with 24% of those who had the psychodynamic treatment. *Mentalization*, developed by Anthony Bateman and Peter Fonagy in the United Kingdom, is a different form of psychodynamic treatment that aims to improve people's capacity to understand their own and other people's mental states, in order to make relationships and emotions more stable. It has been shown to be superior to standard clinical care in reducing hospital admissions, self-harm, and suicide attempts.[33] *Dialectical behavior therapy*, developed by Marsha Linehan in Seattle, is a further type of CBT that focuses on helping individuals develop skills of interpersonal and emotional regulation, as well as increasing their tolerance of distress. It has been shown to be effective in reducing suicide attempts and self-harm.[34]

Antisocial personality disorder is characterized by a pervasive pattern of disregard for, and violation of, other people's rights. There is much less research on the treatment of antisocial personality disorder, and most studies have focused on people who have committed crimes and are in the prison system. Cognitive behavioral group therapy has been shown to reduce reoffending rates and is recommended by NICE.

Alcoholism and Drug Addiction

Alcohol Dependence

For people who are seriously dependent on alcohol, the first thing is to help them to have a period when they do not drink. But from quite early on they also need psychological treatment (usually based on CBT) to help them to remain abstinent and cope with associated problems.

To undergo assisted alcohol withdrawal, those who are most ill need inpatient treatment. But these are a minority, and most people can be treated in the community. The ideal aim is total abstinence, which is facilitated by the use of a benzodiazepine (to reduce the withdrawal symptoms) and acamprosate or naltrexone (to reduce the risk of relapse). But only about a third of those treated this way are still abstinent after a year.[35] A further 30% are improved to some extent. This points to the huge importance of psychological therapy to run in parallel with programs of withdrawal from alcohol. NICE recommends three specific approaches.[36] One is motivational interviewing, which is an intervention that aims to increase an individual's motivation to make changes in their life. A second is behavioral couples therapy, which can help a couple work together to overcome an individual's alcohol dependence. The third is cognitive behavior therapy focused on both drinking and any underlying psychological problems.

A totally different approach is that of Alcoholics Anonymous. Their method relies on the power of support from other members of the group (mutual aid). At each weekly meeting every member introduces himself and acknowledges that he is an alcoholic who is powerless over alcohol. Each new member works through the Twelve-Step Program in which he (or she) recognizes the harm he is causing himself and others, and the need for total abstinence. He acknowledges that he has lost the power to control himself and hands that role to his Higher Power, however conceived. The program is remarkably successful for those who engage with it, although it has not been subjected to rigorous clinical trials.

Drug Dependence

The treatment of drug dependence is similar to that for alcohol. The first step is to bring some order into the person's life. Since drugs like heroin are very expensive, addicts may turn to theft to fund their dependency. The first step toward stabilizing heroin addicts is to provide them with the high that they demand, free of charge. For the worst street addicts, Switzerland and Germany provide comprehensive clinics that initially provide free heroin injections when necessary, but then methadone or buprenorphine, linked to psychosocial support.[37] Britain is trialing free heroin,[38] but the standard NICE-recommended therapy is methadone or buprenorphine.

The ultimate aim must be total abstinence, which is helped by taking naltrexone (to reduce craving). The best residential clinics achieve 40% rates of abstinence after one year. But again, psychological therapy should be a standard component, once the drug situation is under control. The psychological therapy takes three forms. Contingency management is used to reduce drug taking and to promote engagement with services. If the drug user has a nonusing partner, behavioral couples therapy can be helpful as a way of strengthening the way in which the couple can work together to overcome the drug problem. When underlying mental health problems with depression, anxiety, and other conditions are detected, the relevant evidence-based psychological treatment for each condition should also be offered.[39]

Unfortunately, most drug addicts get treatment far too late, partly because taking drugs is illegal. This makes it impossible to treat drug addiction properly. People are frightened to seek help, since it involves admitting to a crime. Moreover, if people are caught, they get a criminal record that makes it much more difficult to get a job[40]—a key step toward improved mental health.

It is vital to decriminalize the use of drugs. This was done in 2001 in Portugal, where people caught with drugs are now sent to a civil tribunal that refers addicts for treatment.[41] As a result the number of people injecting heroin has halved and there has been no increase in general drug use compared with the neighboring country of Spain. Every country should learn from the example of Portugal, and the Czech Republic, which has also decriminalized drug use. This does not mean legalizing the selling of dangerous drugs.

But it would be sensible to allow the regulated supply of less dangerous drugs like cannabis and ecstasy—with proper labeling, information, and testing of products. This would separate the markets for less dangerous drugs from those for heroin and cocaine, and encourage those seeking highs to obtain them in the least dangerous possible way.[42]

Patient Choice

Although there have been enormous advances in the development of effective psychological therapies, there is currently no mental health condition in which a single therapy works for everyone. Given this point, it is important to identify who is likely to benefit from a particular treatment. One of the most consistent findings is that a treatment is more likely to be effective if a person finds it credible and expects to improve.[43] This finding means that therapists need to work hard to ensure that they provide their patients with a clear rationale for treatment. It also suggests that when several different treatments are known to be similarly effective on average, better outcomes are likely to be obtained for individuals if they are allowed to choose the treatment they find most credible.

Recent research has provided some support for this idea. In a randomized controlled trial of treatments for chronic depression, the average result was that after twelve weeks of treatment people were equally likely to respond to CBT or antidepressants. However, those people who initially expressed a preference for CBT did better if they received CBT than if they received medication. And those who preferred medication did better if that was the treatment they got.

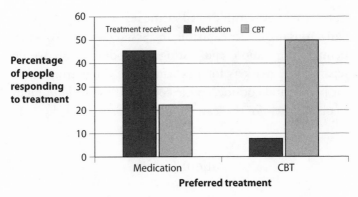

Figure 10.3. People do better on their preferred treatment.

Figure 10.3 shows this striking result.[44] It really matters if people get the treatment they want.

Properly Trained Therapists

Psychological therapies are complex. For them to be effective, they need to be delivered properly. Unless therapists are carefully trained, there will be considerable variability in the competence with which a treatment is delivered. One study found that almost half of the differences between patients in how much they improved with therapy was due to differences in the competence with which their therapist delivered the treatment.[45] Unfortunately, many health care systems have not yet come to terms with this point. In England, for example, a recent national survey of psychological therapies found that more than 30% of people who delivered certain therapies were not trained to do so. Clearly, this needs to change.

To conclude, we have outlined what we currently know about the psychological treatments that work for different mental health conditions. For some conditions (depression, anxiety disorders, PTSD, and bulimia), we have treatments that lead to sustained recovery in half or more people, with many others seeing worthwhile improvements. The treatments that are most effective are generally those that focus on the psychological processes that are known to maintain the condition, rather than on the original cause. For other conditions (schizophrenia, personality disorders, alcoholism, and drug addiction) the benefits of the best treatments are also very worthwhile.

As psychotherapy research goes from strength to strength, more and better therapies will be discovered. In the next few years some current treatments that have not yet been shown to be effective will probably prove their worth. But we already have proven therapies that could benefit millions of people. So can we afford to provide them?

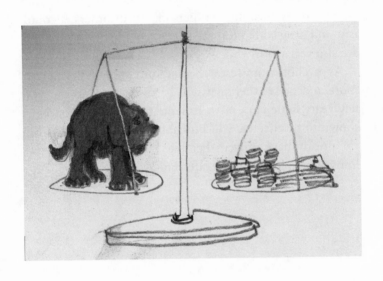

11 ∗ Can We Afford More Therapy?

Nothing astonishes men so much as common sense.

Ralph Waldo Emerson, "Art"

Depression and anxiety can be treated effectively, yet under a third of those affected are in treatment. Surely this is wrong. But the numbers involved are huge, so can we possibly afford the cost of getting help to all who need it?

The answer is a resounding "Yes." First, we do not even ask the question when it comes to chronic physical illnesses like diabetes, lung problems, heart problems, or arthritis. These chronic conditions affect about a third of the whole adult population in advanced countries, and the vast majority of those people get help. The same should hold for people with depression and anxiety disorders, which are often more disabling. But second, there is a remarkable economic fact—that it would cost us nothing (in net terms) to treat all these people. The treatment will generate enough savings to pay for the treatment. That is what this chapter is about.

Savings on Physical Health Care

The first set of savings is on physical health care. As we have seen, whatever their physical health, people who are depressed or anxious go to the hospital more often (as inpatients, outpatients, or for emergency care), and they also go more often to their primary care physician. But, pari passu, when their mental state improves, they use less physical health care. So how does the use of physical health care change when people are given psychological therapy?

Clearly the biggest effects will be found when psychological therapy is given to patients who also have a chronic physical illness. As table 11.1 shows, there is a huge overlap between mental illness and "long-standing physical complaints." People with chronic physical illness account for some 70% of all health care costs.[1] And those of them who have a mental health problem cost some 50% more than other patients with the same physical condition at the same level of severity.[2] So it is not surprising that addressing their mental health can save a great deal of money.

There have been many studies of how physical health care costs alter when people with physical illnesses are also given psychological treatments for their mental health problems. A meta-analysis of ninety-one such studies showed that on average the psychological treatments reduced annual physical health care costs by 20%.[3] In addition, in all but two of the twenty-eight studies where data were available on the cost of psychological treatments, the physical health care savings exceeded the cost of the psychological treatment.

These are US studies. English calculations come to the same conclusion—that treating people for depression or anxiety disorders saves more money for the health services than it costs them. In England such treatment is provided through a program called Improving Access to Psychological Therapies discussed in the next chapter. This includes a range of treatments from low to high intensity, costing on average around $1,000.[4] The average person with physical health problems and mental health problems together costs the health service $9,000 a year in physical health care. So,

Table 11.1. Out of 100 adults, how many have physical complaints, mental illness, or both?

	Have mental illness	Have no mental illness	Total
Have physical complaint(s)	10	32	42
Have no physical complaint	7.5	50.5	58
Total	17.5	82.5	100

if psychological therapy cuts that cost by 20%, the savings are nearly $1,800—much more than the original cost of the psychological treatment.

There is direct evidence that this is the case. One enterprising general practice has followed up 203 of its patients who had been referred to the Improving Access to Psychological Therapies (IAPT) program. It looked at how England's National Health Service costs had changed between the period before referral and two years later. Some of the patients had in the event received no IAPT treatment, some had had partial treatment, and some had had full IAPT treatment. By comparing each of these groups with other patients having the same mix of physical conditions it was possible to estimate how IAPT treatment had affected their usage of physical health care. The answer was that annual physical health care expenditure had fallen by $1,600 as a result of full treatment and $750 for partial treatment—savings big enough to pay for the treatment.[5]

Specific Physical Health Problems

Savings can be especially high when the psychological treatment is adjusted to the specific physical condition of the patient. Here are some examples. Patients with severe *breathing problems* are prone to panic. They feel they may choke to death. In 2006 a London hospital established a cognitive behavioral breathlessness clinic for these patients. One group was treated at once, and the others, randomly selected, were put on a waiting list. The clinic provided four 2-hour sessions of group therapy at weekly intervals.

To evaluate the results, they compared those treated with those not treated, looking at how each group used the health service in the six months before the treatment and in the six months after it. This showed that after treatment those who had been treated went to emergency departments in the hospital 50% less than they would otherwise have done, and spent a third less time in the hospital. Altogether the savings over those six months were $2,000 per person. The clinic had cost only $450 per person, so the savings exceeded the costs by a factor of 4.[6]

Or take the *coronary heart disease* known as angina. Patients with refractory angina are highly prone to both depression and anxiety, including self-defeating safety behaviors like lack of exercise. In 1997 a Liverpool clinic introduced a brief cognitive behavioral program for all these angina patients.[7] This involved two 2-hour interviews eight weeks apart with two consultants (in cardiology and pain management), plus stress-management advice, relaxation tapes, self-help manuals, and graded exercise. In the year after participating in this program, the patients spent 33% fewer days in the hospital than in the year before, as figure 11.1 shows. And fewer of them died. The total saving in cost per patient per year was $3,000—which more than repaid the cost of the intervention.[8]

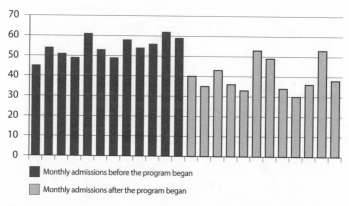

Figure 11.1. A CBT program reduced hospital admissions for refractory angina.

Or consider a Swedish trial of patients discharged from the hospital following treatment for a heart attack.[9] One set of patients was given group CBT in twenty sessions over a year, the other was given none. Figure 11.2 shows the impact of the therapy on those who received it, compared with the control group. It is a striking effect.[10]

That study did not measure the resulting cost savings. But in one US study that did, depressed patients with acute coronary syndrome were randomized between usual care and usual care plus treatment for depression (psychotherapy and/or medication, as the patient chose). Over the following six months, the people who were treated for their depression cost $1,000 less in physical health care.[11]

Finally we can look at *diabetes*. A large American prepaid health plan called the Group Health Cooperative took a group of patients who had diabetes but were also depressed. A randomly selected half of the patients were given specialist care for their depression, while the other half had treatment

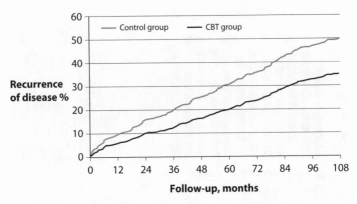

Figure 11.2. CBT reduces the recurrence of cardiovascular disease.
All readings are adjusted for initial medical condition. Cumulative first recurrent fatal and nonfatal cardiovascular events during 9 years (108 months) from baseline, adjusted for the influence of age, sex, marital status, education, smoking habits, co-morbidity, and numerous other medical measures at outset.

as usual. From when the experiment began to twenty-four months later the total health care costs for those treated for depression were $1,100 less per person. Here too the extra cost of the treatment had more than paid for itself.[12]

This evidence has enormous implications. The rationing of mental health care should cease. Making proper evidence-based psychological treatments available in the right dosage is a no-brainer. It will cost the health care system (that is, the insurer) nothing.

Savings on Welfare

There is also a major second saving—to the welfare system. Mental illness, unlike physical illness, is mainly a problem for people of working age. By stopping so many people from working, mental health problems cost the community billions in welfare benefits and lost taxes. Treating these conditions successfully can lead to huge financial savings, which fully repay the cost of the treatment.

The mechanism is simple. Making treatment available can help distressed people to stay in work. And if they are out of work it can help them back into work by giving them the psychological strength and confidence to face the labor market. In fact, even a course of group CBT for unemployed people has been shown to double the numbers who find work.[13]

We can put some numbers on the savings. Suppose we treat 100 typical people with depression and anxiety disorders (some working, some not). From the available evidence we can expect that over the next 25 months at least 4 of the 100 people treated will work who would not otherwise have done so. That makes altogether at least 100 extra months at work and off welfare benefits (4 x 25). Averaged over the 100 people treated, that amounts to at least one month off benefits per person treated. The resulting savings on welfare benefits and lost taxes are at least as much as the cost of the therapy.[14] This is true in both the United States and Britain. Thus the cost of the therapy is covered twice over—in these savings as well as in reduced physical health care.

But how robust is the 4% assumption about the effects of therapy on employment?[15] A randomized trial in the United States followed up patients who had received cognitive therapy for depression over a two-year period. By the end of that time 18% more were in work than otherwise would have been. (By contrast patients allocated to antidepressant medication for the same two-year period had no significant

extra employment, nor did those allocated to pill placebo.[16])
This 18% is a very large effect. In another randomized trial
of "enhanced mental health treatment" for depression, the
effect over twelve months was 5 percentage points—again
bigger than we have assumed in our calculation.[17]

Likewise, when a group of patients with general anxiety
disorder or panic attacks were given "collaborative mental health care," their employment rate twelve months later
was up by 16 percentage points compared with treatment
as usual. And their absenteeism rate was down by the equivalent of thirty-one days a year. Both of these impacts are
much bigger than we have allowed for.[18]

The only British randomized trial of employment effects
is the one we have already referred to. It covers some three
hundred long-term unemployed people. One group had
seven weeks of group CBT, in sessions lasting three hours
each. The other group had an equal number of sessions of
generalized social support. After four months, over twice as
many of the CBT group had found full-time work—34%,
compared with 13% for the others.[19]

There is also another way to get a handle on how treatment affects employment. This involves two steps: first, the
effect of treatment on recovery, and then the effect of recovery on employment. Looking at it that way gives even more
encouraging estimates of the overall effect of treatment on
employment.[20]

Unfortunately, patients treated in the new English program for Improving Access to Psychological Therapies have
not been followed long enough to confirm the 4% assumption. But the number who shift off benefit during the brief
period of treatment is extremely encouraging.[21] There is
every reason to suppose that the government's savings on

welfare benefits and lost taxes exceed the full cost of wider access to psychological therapy.

Moreover, from the standpoint of the citizen it is not only the financial burden on government funds that matters. There is also a wider question: what are the benefits to society as a whole? This is the standard question in social cost-benefit analysis. In this case the costs of treatment are the same as before. These are "real resource costs" and they need to be compared with the "real economic benefits" that result. Savings on benefit payments and taxes are not a real benefit to the economy as a whole, since the state saves the money but the recipient loses the money. The real economic benefit is the extra output that is produced by having more people at work. This is whatever is produced by an average of one extra month of work per person. This is much bigger than the cost of having someone on welfare benefits. So the output gains greatly exceed the cost of the treatment. And even more can be achieved if therapy for those out of work is accompanied by vigorous efforts to place people in work.

Conclusion

We have here a double whammy. The costs of the psychological therapy are covered twice over. They are covered by savings on physical health care, and they are also covered by the government's savings on welfare. At the same time there is a massive reduction in human suffering.

From 2004 onward England's NICE was recommending that all patients with depression or anxiety disorders be offered evidence-based psychological therapy. But by 2007 not more than 3% of people in England with these conditions were getting therapy (and usually it was not the therapy NICE recommended).[22] According to Sir Mike Rawlins, when he was chairman of NICE, this was a case of scandalous disregard—by far the greatest disregard of any of NICE's guidelines. At the same time it was an economic nonsense. The time was ripe to expose the outrage and to argue for a radical new initiative.

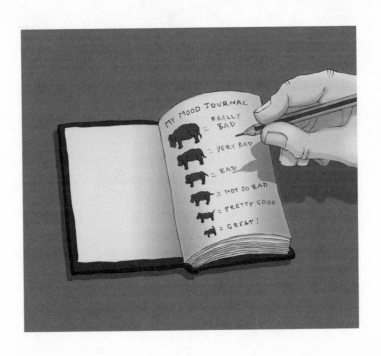

12 * Improving Access to Psychological Therapies

We will build a groundbreaking psychological therapy service in England.

Alan Johnson, Secretary of State for Health, 2008

Despite all the evidence for psychological therapy, most people with depression and anxiety disorders in most countries are not offered it. If anything, they are offered pills. But three-quarters of them would prefer psychological therapy.[1] How can this be provided?

One possible answer comes from a radical new development in England. It is called Improving Access to Psychological Therapies and has come to be known as IAPT. This is a systematic way of organizing the delivery of evidence-based psychological therapy within England's National Health Service. It aims to provide, in every locality, teams of well-trained therapists working under expert supervision. The progress of each patient is measured session by session, which helps both therapist and patient to advance the treatment. It also, crucially, tells those who fund the service whether they are getting value for money. In fact everything about the system (other than patient identity) is transparent.[2] Anyone who is interested can access the performance of every service as well as all the operating documents of the program: the skills required of each type of therapist, the training curricula, the guidelines for supervisors, and the guidelines for commissioners.

IAPT has been something of an infant prodigy. It only started in late 2008, but by 2013 it was treating some 400,000 people a year, nearly half of whom had recovered by the end of treatment. Since the model has worked so well and is so transparent, it has generated major interest in other countries. Interest has come from at least seven countries, and Norway and Sweden have already started to introduce their own version of the system.

In England, IAPT is still only halfway to what is required if everyone who wants help is to be offered it. But enough has been achieved to ask, how did it happen? how well has it done? and how is it structured?

The IAPT Story

In Britain there are two key moments when you can inject new ideas into public policy—one is before a general election and the other is before the government's periodic "spending reviews." Our story revolves around these moments.

In 2005 there was to be a general election, and the Labour government was writing its election manifesto. This was a real opportunity to raise the profile of psychological therapy. So we wrote a paper for Tony Blair's Policy Unit called "Mental Health: Britain's Biggest Social Problem?"[3]

This argued that to implement the NICE guidelines we should be able to treat at least 15% of the diagnosable population each year, and this would require some 8,000 more therapists in England, most of whom would have to be trained.

The paper made its impact through three simple points. The first was the scale of suffering and the injustice of denying people the evidence-based treatments they preferred. Second (and very important) there was the economic argument, that mental illness cost the government billions of pounds, and treatment would therefore have no net cost to the Treasury. And third, routine outcome measurement would show what the system was really achieving. Initially, the proposed development would concentrate on adults (but only because there is more evidence there than for children).

Blair's Policy Unit responded by organizing a Downing Street seminar where we put forward our arguments. Many of those present expressed their amazement that psychological therapy had now become so scientifically validated. The impact was considerable. A few months later Labour's election manifesto included a commitment to "improve our services for people with mental health problems at primary and secondary levels, including behavioral as well as drug therapies."[4]

Labour won the election and a program was established for Improving Access to Psychological Therapies. But at that stage there was no clear view of what the program should consist of. One school of thought favored little more than a bit more counseling, and there was originally to be only one pilot site (Doncaster), focused on low-intensity therapy such as guided self-help. Under pressure, a second site (Newham in east London) was established, weighted more to high-intensity therapy. That was one step in the right direction. A second came when the Department of Health set up a group of experts to advise the program, and they too pressed for a more broad-based approach.

At the same time we formed a Mental Health Policy Group at the London School of Economics that worked out the key steps needed to get from here to where we wanted to be, over a period of six years.[5] A new service had to be established with its own standards and its own way of working. This could only be done well by advancing unevenly, area by area, and establishing one high-quality service after another. Each new service had to be good enough to provide placements for the new trainees.

The next question was, "Is there any new money available for this program?" From on high the answer was "No." But it was obvious that unless a plan was produced for what was desirable, the program would get nowhere. The courageous civil servant in charge of mental health gave the go-ahead for that approach.

However, as the October 2007 spending review approached, things did not look good. A Treasury committee of officials reported that the plan was not based on evidence and was also too expensive. But then things changed. Gordon Brown became Prime Minister, and he and his Downing Street officials backed the program. At the same time an outstanding politician, Alan Johnson, was appointed Secretary of State for Health. On October 10, 2007, World Mental Health Day, he made his announcement:

> We will build a groundbreaking psychological therapy service in England. Backed by new investment rising to £170 million by 2010–11, the service will be capable of treating 900,000 additional patients suffering from depression and anxiety over the next three years. Around half are likely to be completely cured, with

many fewer people with mental health problems having to depend on sick pay and benefits.

And he provided every penny that had been asked for. (By "treating" he meant seeing at least once, including assessment and advice. The recovery rate would apply to those who have a course of therapy, that is, who are seen two or more times.)

So that was the plan—to roll out a new service nationwide that could make the NICE-recommended therapies available to everybody who needed them. It would take six years to do it, though detailed commitments were only made for the first three years (the period of the spending review). By 2015 the aim was to employ some 8,000 therapists in England—roughly forty for a typical population of quarter of a million people. Of these some 6,000 therapists would have to be trained—IAPT was creating a whole new profession of psychological therapists using evidence-based therapy. Given the shortage of CBT therapists in particular, and CBT's proven effectiveness, most of the training would initially be in CBT, but would cover other therapies later. So the aim was for steady expansion, involving more and more areas, till the whole country was covered within six years.

Following the announcement, the next year was one of fevered activity.[6] Competencies had to be identified for treating each particular disorder in the way NICE had recommended.[7] National training curricula were developed for one-year courses, involving two days a week in college and three days of supervised practice;[8] the curricula focused on the particular evidence-based treatment shown to be effective for the specific type of anxiety or depression. That done, colleges competed to participate. At the same time local services were also competing to be part of the first wave of services. Services had to show they could provide the trainees with patients who had the conditions they had been trained to treat—plus competent supervisors.[9] The whole activity was coordinated by a small team in the Department of Health with a brilliant administrator, working closely with at least thirty professionals from the field.

In September 2008 some thirty-five services opened, covering about a quarter of the country, and about 1,000 trainees began their training. Every year since then has seen a further expansion of services, and by 2014 they had reached three-quarters of their planned capacity for 2015. In the first six years, over 6,000 therapists had completed IAPT training courses.[10]

All this was achieved despite another election in 2010 and another spending review. In that election, for the first time, every major political party included psychological therapy in its manifesto.[11] And after the election, the new coalition government's spending review strongly endorsed the program and expanded it to cover children, people with comorbid physical conditions, and those with severe mental illness. The funding was to increase each year by the same amount as under Labour, and by year six the program was to receive £340 million a year.

However, from the third year onward this finance has ceased to be ring-fenced. Local commissioners receive a block grant that includes the IAPT money as a component, but local commissioners then make their own decisions about how to spend their total grant. Some have spent more than was allocated in the block grant and some less. Up to 2012 the aggregate spending was much as planned. But from 2012 the program suffered seriously from the reorganization of the National Health Service's administrative structures. Skilled commissioners departed and many services were left unsure about their ability to continue expanding. There was a loss of momentum. However, the reorganization is now complete. All political parties are committed to the ongoing expansion of IAPT, and it is happening.

Measuring Outcomes

To know whether IAPT is a success, we need to be able to measure whether people get better. Traditionally mental health services have not been good at measuring outcomes. Before IAPT started fewer than 40% of the people in England who received psychological therapy had an objective measure of their symptoms at the beginning and end of therapy.[12] Furthermore, there was reason to suppose that when therapy services had a lot of missing data they tended to overestimate how well they were doing, because people who failed to provide data tended to have done less well.[13] Clearly, if the National Health Service was to make a major investment in IAPT, an improved system for collecting outcomes was required. The traditional system asked patients to complete questionnaires twice: at the beginning of therapy and at the last session. It failed because many people end therapy at a different time from when their therapist expects. The solution was to move to a session-by-session outcome monitoring system in which patients are asked to complete a simple measure of their symptoms at every session, ensuring that an end of treatment symptom score is almost always available. This system gave the therapist a much better idea of how the patient was progressing. It has also enabled IAPT to record and publish[14] the clinical outcomes of 97% of people who have a course of therapy.[15] This is a remarkable achievement that ensures we really know how well the services are doing.

People Get Better

What has been achieved so far? A large number of people have already been treated. Table 12.1 shows some basic figures. (Remember that England is a country of some fifty-three million people.) The first row shows the numbers who had at least one encounter with the service. IAPT was conceived as an assessment *and* treatment service. It was always thought that a significant proportion of people would benefit from just an assessment and advice. Others would need a formal course of therapy. The numbers seen are broadly in line with what was originally planned.[16] About 40% of those have a single session. The rest go on to receive a course of therapy involving at least two sessions. In 2014 nearly 400,000 were treated in this way.

About 46% of people who had a course of treatment recovered, and around two-thirds showed systematic improvement.[17] From clinical trials a reasonable expectation is that 50% of those diagnosable should recover, and that was the target Alan Johnson set for IAPT. Recovery rates have been somewhat below this level, but they are rising, and are quite impressive if we allow for the high proportion of therapy still being delivered by trainees or very newly qualified staff.

The IAPT approach achieves seriously good results for people who have been ill for years and even decades. This

Table 12.1. What has IAPT achieved?

	2008/9	2009/10	2010/11	2011/12	2012/13	2013/14
Numbers seen	40,000	180,000	380,000	530,000	600,000	720,000
Numbers treated	10,000	90,000	250,000	330,000	380,000	395,000
Recovery rate (%)		38	39	44	46	46

emerged clearly from the pilots in Doncaster and Newham where data were collected on how long the patients had been depressed or anxious. The average time across the two sites was three and a half years, and over two-thirds of the people had been anxious or depressed for more than six months. If we look only at this "chronic" group, the recovery rates at both sites were 52%, which compares with the figure of under 20% that would have been expected from natural recovery.[18] Moreover, when patients were followed up nine months later most of these gains had been maintained.[19]

The most obvious failure of IAPT so far is the huge variation of performance in different parts of the country.[20] This applies not only to access, but also to recovery rates. One would expect some variation in access when a program is being rolled out in sequence across the country. But recovery rates should not vary as much as they do in figure 12.1.

There is however a silver lining to the chart—it shows how well IAPT can do when it is done well. By 2014 a quarter of the areas in England had already exceeded the national target of 50% recovery, and some were reporting consistent recovery rates of over 60%.[21] Clearly, the next step is to identify the factors associated with success and help

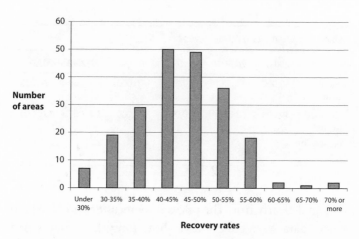

Figure 12.1. Recovery rates vary greatly between areas (IAPT 2014).

poorer performing services to use this information to improve their outcomes.

So far there have been several approaches to finding out what works best. Each has been informative. One involved analyzing the data collected in the first year of the IAPT program to identify characteristics of services with particularly high recovery rates. The results were highly instructive.[22] The closer the IAPT model described below is followed, the higher the recovery rates. Recovery is higher where there are more highly trained and experienced therapists. It is also higher where patients receive more sessions—to achieve 50% recovery rates a service needs to provide an average of at least eight sessions per person, with many individuals receiving more sessions. Recovery is higher where there are good step-up rates to high-intensity treatment when low-intensity has failed.[23] And recovery is higher when patients are treated according to NICE guidelines. This was evident for both high- and low-intensity therapy. At high intensity, NICE recommends for mild to moderate depression both CBT and counseling, and the two treatments did equally well. However, for generalized anxiety disorder, NICE recommends CBT but not counseling, and recovery rates were significantly higher with CBT. At low intensity, NICE recommends for depression guided self-help, but not self-help without guidance; guided self-help did better. Finally, recovery rates are higher the larger the service—there is real value from a comprehensive and well-led organization.

Another approach involved reviewing with clinicians the treatment of every person who was discharged from a large service during a one-month period without having recovered. The review identified several themes that prompted service reorganizations. In the year prior to the review, recovery rates averaged 45%. Afterward they immediately rose to 65% and have stayed at that level. Interestingly, the therapies the service and the staff offered did not change. The improvements were achieved by ensuring that patients started at the right place in the stepped care system, were stepped up promptly if necessary, had a choice of therapies, and received an adequate number of sessions.[24]

To help IAPT services learn from each other, a public website[20] has been created that displays in an accessible format detailed performance information about each service. Clinicians in the services are encouraged to benchmark their service against neighbors and to develop collaborative networks that share clinically useful information and procedures.

Finally, the Department of Health has convened workshops in which the highest performing services are invited to share their top tips. A consistent theme is the importance of strong clinical leadership that is focused on patient recovery, uses the data to identify and test innovations in patient care, and provides therapists with feedback on their individual recovery rates in a supportive manner. Therapists are also given the opportunity to regularly update their skills in service-sponsored continuing professional development events.

So IAPT has shown that it is possible in a short time to make big improvements in the lives of hundreds of thousands of people. That is why other countries are looking to the IAPT model for insight into how they might handle this major human problem.

The IAPT Model

What exactly is the IAPT model? There are six main criteria a service has to satisfy if it is to be an IAPT service.

- It has to deliver only evidence-based, NICE-recommended therapies.[25] This includes not only CBT but interpersonal therapy, brief psychodynamic therapy, couples therapy, and counseling for depression.
- It has to employ therapists who are fully trained in how to deliver the relevant treatment.
- It has to measure patient outcomes on a session-by-session basis, with at least 90% completeness of data.[26]
- Each patient receives a professional assessment when she arrives and is then allocated to high- or low-intensity treatment, as appropriate. About 46% get low intensity only, 34% get high intensity only, and 20% get both—

having been stepped up to high intensity after low intensity failed.[27]

- Each therapist must have weekly supervision, and each trainee must have a well-qualified supervisor.
- The service must be open to patients who refer themselves, without going through their general practitioner (GP). This breaks with all normal arrangements in the National Health Service. When it was proposed, some people argued that it would attract the "worried well." On the contrary, it was found that patients who self-refer are as ill as those coming through their GP. They have also been ill longer, and recover as well (often with fewer sessions, reflecting their high level of motivation). They also include a higher proportion of people from black and minority ethnic groups than patients referred by GPs, and this helps to ensure that IAPT patients have a more similar ethnic balance to the population at large.[28]

Thus IAPT is a system, and it involves a team of people with different skills able to handle the range of problems that people bring. But it is not a clinic in an ivory tower. It aims to treat everyone as near as possible to their home in the most acceptable setting possible—such as the premises of a GP practice, a voluntary organization, or a community mental health team.

It is in fact a hub-and-spoke model. There is a central office where the clinical director and chief administrator work, and where there are rooms for supervision, training, keeping patients' records, and the telephone support for guided self-help. But most of the face-to-face therapy is given much nearer to where the patients live, and in close contact with the patient's doctor. Wherever the therapy happens, all the therapists are part of the IAPT team, and are appointed and supervised by IAPT.

So, you might ask, why not get the primary care practices (GPs) to employ their own therapists? The answer is quality control. Therapists need to be supervised by senior therapists. If they are to develop as professionals, that needs to be their identity. They need an employer who can properly judge their performance, and a system that offers a proper prospect of career progression.

Alternatively, you might say, why are they not simply a part of the existing "secondary" specialist mental health service that runs inpatient and community mental health services? The problem here is that due to scarcity of funds these services have had to focus heavily on psychotic and ex-psychotic patients. That is where their heart lies, and that is one reason why in every country there has been such appalling neglect of people with the much more common conditions of depression and anxiety disorder.

Even so, in many cases the IAPT contract has in fact gone to a secondary care provider. But in every case IAPT has its independent structure and its own administrator and lead psychological therapist. That is what has enabled it to develop with confidence, as a separate entity.

Some patients are of course too complex for IAPT to handle, and they are then referred to secondary care services that often include psychiatrists. So why, you might ask, does IAPT employ only psychological therapists and no psychiatrists? It is a fair question. As IAPT becomes increasingly involved with patients with physical as well as mental symptoms, it will surely develop more complex relationships both with psychiatrists and with specialists in chronic

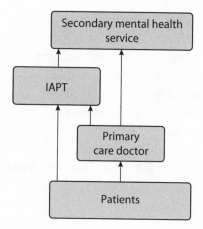

Figure 12.2. Where IAPT fits in.

physical illness. But one thing is sure: IAPT would never have been so successful if it had not been an autonomous service, able to develop an ethos and standards of its own.

As figure 12.2 shows, IAPT is not part of primary care or secondary care—it lies in between. That is vital. And it can be accessed through self-referral without going to the family doctor.

Finally, how do these IAPT services come into being? They are commissioned by the local commissioners, through whom the funding for the National Health Service flows.[29] Generally, commissioning is done by open tender once every three years or so, and providers who bid may be secondary mental health trusts (most commonly) but also voluntary organizations, and sometimes private sector providers. To qualify, a provider has to satisfy the criteria we described earlier. The service is then subject to regular outside appraisal, more detailed if the service is taking trainees. And most important it has to supply (anonymized) data on every patient treated, in order that we can know what access it provides and how successfully its patients are treated—do they actually recover? This outcome measurement is probably the most important single feature of IAPT. It is really the only ultimate guarantee of quality. The people who commission mental health services are always tempted to save money by dumbing down quality. But if they do this, they will get found out—it will be revealed in the published outcome figures. In fact, providing services and the public with information on outcomes is key to the future of mental health in England.

The Critics of IAPT

Even so, IAPT, like everything human, has its critics. Some of the complaints are justified, since what happens locally on the ground never corresponds exactly to what its originators intended. For example, there have been commissioners who have limited the number of sessions of treatment a person can receive initially to six or less. This is an outrage. It is as if a commissioner said to a surgeon, "We will pay for a one-hour operation and if it is not finished after sixty minutes, sew the patient up and we will consider whether to let you continue treatment." This kind of situation is not the fault of IAPT but of the commissioners, and IAPT has achieved whatever it has despite being sometimes driven off course from outside. In some ways it is a miracle that so much has been achieved.

Moreover, some of the criticisms that are made are really quite misleading. For example, some people say that IAPT only provides CBT, but in fact it provides a range of

NICE-recommended therapies. As of today around 38% of all the high-intensity therapists employed in IAPT describe themselves as either counselors or therapists from non-CBT therapies.[30] But IAPT is of course confined to therapies recommended by NICE, and that is the biggest ground for complaint.

As a matter of history, however, the expansion of psychological therapy would never have happened at all without NICE. Policy makers these days demand evidence before spending taxpayers' money, especially if the area of spending lies outside their comfort zone. It was NICE's evidence that forced them to act. This does not mean that NICE is the last word. There must be other good therapies that could prove themselves if properly trialed, and we must make sure there is financing to make this possible.

But has IAPT worked to the detriment of psychological therapy in other parts of the National Health Service? On occasions it has, but not in general. As figure 12.3 shows, non-IAPT expenditure on psychological therapy (largely in secondary mental health) has not in fact shrunk. Instead, expenditure on psychological therapy in the National Health Service has doubled as a share of mental health spending: a substantial achievement.

Another criticism concerns the motivation for IAPT. Is it basically a program to push people into work? Not at all. It is a great humanitarian project, just like any other major health program. It is also convenient that, when more patients work, this saves the state money. But this is not the point of the program, and, as we have said, it only involves a small fraction of patients (we talked earlier about 4%). The program is for all who suffer, whether work is an issue for them or not.

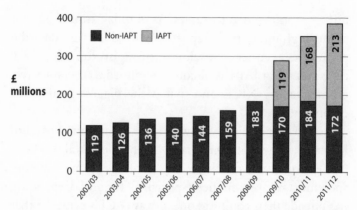

Figure 12.3. Expenditure on psychological therapy has risen sharply (England).

Finally, some critics have argued that IAPT greatly exaggerates its recovery rates.[31] These rates take the person's score when they are first seen and compare it with their score when they are last seen. Such a calculation can only be made for people who are seen twice or more. The critics have two arguments. First they say that those who recover on this measure should be expressed as a proportion of everyone who is referred to IAPT even if they are never seen or seen only once. This is like saying that we should assess the success of surgery by looking at everyone referred to a surgeon, whether or not they receive surgery, and then see what proportion of those originally referred have a successful operation. It is a mad approach, but sadly these misleading analyses get reported.

A more reasonable critique is that patients have not been followed by the services to see that they remain as well as patients do in randomized controlled trials. Commissioners have not been keen to support the cost of this follow-up; however, we hope this will change in the future. The sustained improvement that was seen at Newham and Doncaster is encouraging, but these results need to be confirmed in every service. The ideal would be if patients finishing IAPT therapy were to complete the IAPT measures the next time they attended their GP practice.

Where Next for IAPT?

IAPT is not more than halfway to where it needs to be. When we proposed the development of IAPT, we thought about what could reasonably be attempted over a six-year period. We judged that, if quality was to be achieved, we could aim within six years at a service that saw each year some 15% of the six million people then suffering from depression and anxiety disorders in England. This would involve some 8,000 therapists, of whom 6,000 would need to be trained by the program. This proved a feasible objective.

But it became increasingly obvious that much more was going to be needed if everyone who needed and wanted psychological therapy was to get it.[32] The most obvious evidence of this was that, although the numbers treated were rising rapidly, *waiting times were unacceptable*. In 2014 20% of new patients had to wait over eight weeks before being seen,[33] and a few had to wait a year or more.

A second major issue was the large number of people with *chronic physical illnesses* (like lung disease, heart disease, arthritis, and diabetes) who are also mentally ill. Increasingly we realized that IAPT had to help more of the four million people who have physical illness accompanied by mental distress. As we have seen, there are powerful ways of doing this, but they involve more than the simplest forms of

CBT. They require the therapist to understand the physical illness, and the fears and despair it gives rise to. In the next phase of IAPT new forms of training and treatment have to be developed to deal with this group of people. And there also has to be closer working between therapists and hospital and family doctors.

A third issue is the treatment of people with *schizophrenia and other near-psychotic problems*. The NICE guidelines say they should be offered psychological therapy, but in most cases they are not. So when in 2011 the new coalition government announced its policies for mental health,[34] it extended the remit of IAPT to include people with comorbid physical illness, and people with schizophrenia and near-psychotic problems, and older people.[35] But it provided no further money, except to support pilot studies.

When the initial phase of IAPT ends in 2015, there will have to be a *major further phase of expansion*. The numbers seen will need to rise from 15% of need to 25% of need by 2020, with the same 50% recovery target. And there will be a *waiting time target* for access to psychological therapy, as there is for specialist physical care: we believe at least 80% should begin their treatment within twenty-eight days. All this will call for the training of at least 1,000 therapists a year.

There is also another major problem that needs addressing: *employment*. For most people work is highly therapeutic. It gives meaning and purpose to life, and a reason to engage with the world each day. But therapists are not experts in how patients can find work or how they can remain in work if they have it. So therapists need to work alongside employment and welfare advisers, whenever that is what their patients need. For this reason IAPT guidelines have always said that each team should include one employment specialist for every eight therapists. Alas, this has not happened, except in a few areas. The reason is of some political interest. Originally the Health Department's proposed budget for IAPT included the money to pay for employment support. But the Department for Work and Pensions said it would like to pay for it. So the money was struck out of the Health budget, but Work and Pensions never found the money themselves. This is a perfect example of why joint funding and joint responsibility for any program should be avoided whenever possible.

In the next phase it is imperative to address this employment issue directly, for the sake of patients and to improve the government's finances. At present only half of all the mentally ill people on disability benefits are in any form of treatment for their condition.[36] This is madness. Taxpayers are supporting people who have a treatable condition, but half of these people are not in treatment. They should automatically be referred to IAPT.[37] But this will only work well if IAPT teams include enough employment advisers.

One last issue—research. IAPT has an unparalleled information base, and therefore extraordinary potential to improve itself through research. As we have seen, recovery rates vary far too much between different services. We can make this knowledge public, and provide research findings that enable the weaker services to improve. These findings will also be highly relevant in any other country that wants to offer a similar service.

IAPT is not perfect. Like any organization, it has unintended side effects. But it has in a short time produced what the eminent psychiatrist Sir Simon Wessely has called "the greatest revolution in British mental health in fifty years."

In most countries adults with depression and anxiety disorders get a raw deal, and the IAPT approach is one way to help them.

The United States and Other Countries

Of course, other countries have also started to grapple with the paradox that highly effective psychological therapies for mental health problems exist but very few people are offered them.

In the United States, the president's New Freedom Commission[38] concluded in 2003 that a transformation of mental health care delivery was required, and particularly noted that evidence-based psychological therapies were poorly implemented and rarely available.[39] The Veterans Health Administration (VHA) responded by developing an ambitious, large-scale implementation program that aimed to intervene at multiple levels.[40] At the policy level it was agreed that all veterans with specific mental health conditions should be offered evidence-based psychological therapies. VHA staff members were offered training in fifteen evidence-based treatments, many of which overlap with those provided in IAPT, and were given ongoing supervision after the end of training, as in IAPT. Local evidence-based practice coordinators were appointed to facilitate implementation in each VHA medical center. Veterans were made more aware of the value of evidence-based psychological therapies, and surveys of progress in local implementation were conducted. By 2013, 6,400 VHA staff members had received training in one or more evidence-based therapies. Recently, the VHA has started to publish in academic journals the outcomes that VHA staff achieved with veterans while staff members were going through the training program. Clear benefits have been observed for veterans with posttraumatic stress disorder,[41] depression,[42] and insomnia.[43] As with IAPT, this impressive program is not without its critics.[44] However, it has achieved a lot in a small amount of time.

Looking at the rest of the world, the Australian government has substantially increased funding for people to be referred for psychological therapy, if their family doctor identifies a mental health problem that would benefit. There is also a drive to make Internet-based cognitive-behavior therapy widely available, not least as a way of reaching people in remote rural locations. In Stockholm an IAPT-like pilot program with a strong emphasis on therapist training, stepped care, and routine outcome monitoring has been established. We understand that other European countries and Canada are watching closely and considering similar initiatives.

Lessons from IAPT

Every country is different and each will need to address the problem of how to increase access to evidence-based psychological therapies in a manner that fits with its local health care systems and economy. However, there are some lessons from the IAPT experience that we feel have general relevance.

The importance of economics. The IAPT program would not have existed without our economic arguments. In most countries there is a debate about the spiraling costs of health care. We argued that better mental health care is an economic no-brainer. The cost of making effective psychological therapies more widely available is more than covered by the savings in physical health care costs and state benefits, and by improvements in workplace productivity and tax revenues. In the United Kingdom the government provides most health care and also receives the range of savings. In countries where insurance companies fund much health care, the insurer will only benefit from the savings in physical health care costs, plus longer-term reductions in mental health care costs. However, as we showed in chapter 11, these are more than enough to justify expanding psychological therapy provision.

Universal outcome monitoring and public transparency. It is clear that insurance organizations, health administrators, and governments also need reliable information on the outcomes that are achieved with an expansion of access to evidence-based psychological therapies. Without such information, it is difficult for them to justify the investment. The session-by-session outcome monitoring used in IAPT provides such information on almost everyone who receives treatment. Therapists also benefit from being able to adjust their treatment plans based on such regular feedback. Publication of outcome data allows services to learn from one another and encourages the public to contribute to local discussions about the commissioning of services.

High-quality therapist training. Much progress is being made in developing new and effective psychological treatments. To ensure these are faithfully delivered to the public, we need to ensure that the psychological therapy workforce is properly trained in the delivery of the treatments, many of which may have been developed after clinicians initially qualified. Such training requires written therapist guides (manuals), the development of national training curricula, specification of the competencies required for each therapy, and assessments of the extent to which the competencies have been acquired.

Therapy services. Traditionally, much public provision of psychological therapy has been provided by talented psychological therapists working in isolation. Such work provides strong patient choice and will continue to be important. However, IAPT has highlighted the additional benefit of organizing some therapy provision within integrated services. The benefits include seamless implementation of stepped care and a guarantee of regular supervision for all therapists. It is interesting that IAPT is beginning to show that substantial improvements in recovery rates can be achieved by thoughtful reorganization of the way in which a stepped-care system is delivered, even when the staff working in a service and the therapies that it provides remain constant.

In all these ways we can deliver much more effective therapy to many more adults. But what about children?

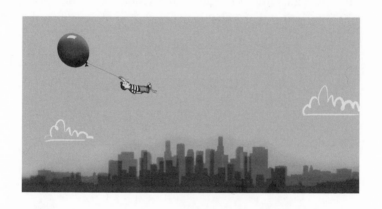

13 * What Works for Young People?

Make me have a mum and dad that love me and to start my horrid life AGAIN and not have so much sadness in my life.

Eight-year-old girl[1]

Nowhere is the gap between rhetoric and performance greater than in how we treat child mental health. A leading British official once said, "For as long as I can remember, services for children have been described as an important priority for the national health service and in the next breath as a Cinderella service—save that this Cinderella has never got near to the ball."[2]

The situation is similar in almost every country. People just do not want to acknowledge the scale of the problem. Yet in the United States and elsewhere roughly one in ten children age five to sixteen would be diagnosed as suffering from a serious mental health problem.[3] The shocking thing is that only a quarter of these children are being helped by specialist mental health services.[4] This is true in Britain, and things are, if anything, rather worse in most other countries.

This is incredibly shortsighted. As we have seen, the majority of children with mental health problems go on to be mentally ill as adults.[5] It would surely be better to treat their condition when it first emerges, rather than to wait till they have wasted years of their life in misery or in destructive behavior. The humanitarian case is obvious, and so is the clinical case—it is easier to deal with most problems before they get too bad.[6]

But there is also a powerful economic case for early intervention—for stopping the stream of damage in its tracks as early as possible. In Britain, someone with conduct disorder in childhood will cost society roughly £150,000 more (in present value terms) than someone without it—mainly due to the costs of criminal justice.[7] The comparable figure in the United States is probably higher, due to the greater frequency of incarceration.[8] But suppose we take the figure of £150,000. It has a very simple implication. If we had a treatment that cost £5,000 per child, it would cost us nothing if it saved only one in thirty of the children. And on top of that come the humanitarian gains.

Do we have effective treatments? In general the answer is yes.[9] Less research has been done on children's problems than adults, but we already have a whole range of effective treatments that are recommended by NICE.[10]

Anxiety and Depression

For anxiety and depression, the recommended treatments are very similar to those for adults. CBT can be successfully used with children from the age of eight upward, either individually or in groups with other children. For anxiety the recovery rate with CBT in randomized trials is 50–60%.[11] For depression, CBT or interpersonal therapy or (in carefully selected cases) medication also produce good recovery rates. Neither psychoanalytic therapy nor counseling have a consistent record of success in trials,[12] so NICE does not recommend them.

Disruptive Behavior

In most countries the biggest, single mental health problem in childhood is conduct disorder—affecting some 5% of all children at any one time. We are talking of such symptoms as tantrums, disobedience, spitefulness, blaming others, theft, and (worse) destructiveness, violence, using weapons, physical cruelty, and running away from home.

Here too effective treatments exist. Except in severe cases the standard treatment for most young children is "parent training"—most commonly the Incredible Years Program developed by Carolyn Webster-Stratton of the University of Washington. Parents are seen for weekly two-hour group sessions for up to sixteen weeks.[13] In the first three weeks they learn how to tune in to their children. Instead of nagging them, they learn how to play with them, letting the child lead the game and just commenting nonjudgmentally on what they are doing. In the next stage they learn how to praise their children, whenever they behave in a desirable way. Only after that comes the setting of rules—how to be authoritative when it is necessary, with firm, clear instructions given full-face with eye contact. The instructions should be as concrete as possible and lead to immediate action. Rewards can be promised but only in terms of "when you do this," not "if you do it." The final sequence is about punishments—again as simple as possible and small enough not to generate despair. Small, attention-seeking naughtiness should be ignored, but the worst offenses should lead to Time Out (5–10 minutes maximum).

This program has been widely trialed and is used in many countries. One of the largest trials is in England. Seven years after being treated, the children were 80% less likely to have oppositional defiant disorder (for which see Brian in chapter 3), compared with those not treated. And, according to parents' reports, their behavior was much improved, compared with reports on other children.[14]

However, the most difficult children need more than training provided to their parent. The children need to be seen themselves—either on their own, or often with their parent. Younger children will be seen with their parent and often treated using the Parent-Child Game, where the parent is taught how to play constructively with their child. Older children benefit increasingly from being seen on their own, as well as with their parents. From age eight onward the content of this "problem-solving therapy" becomes increasingly cognitive. For example, in "anger management" children are taught to observe and manage their emotions, to think before they react to someone else's behavior, to adopt the perspective of the other person, and so on.[15]

For really troubled children there is multisystemic therapy, which involves at least twelve home visits, working with the family as a whole and drawing on a mixture of CBT, parent training, couples therapy, and other structured approaches. Even with the most difficult children good results have been obtained, with only 22% being subsequently arrested, compared with 71% of the children who only received individual treatment.[16]

Some children have the very specific problem known as attention deficit hyperactivity disorder (ADHD). Typically, these children have a combination of three sets of difficulties. Firstly, there is the issue of attention deficit—the inability to concentrate on anything. Secondly, there is hyperactivity: they cannot sit still and are always on the move. Thirdly, these children are impulsive, doing everything in a rush, unable to inhibit, blurting out answers, and so on. This is different from the antisocial behavior seen in conduct disorders. There is a strong genetic and biological element in this problem, and it is perhaps therefore not surprising that it generally responds well to medication. If treated with an amphetamine called methylphenidate (Ritalin), a stimulant that boosts the level of dopamine, 75% of children lose their symptoms.[17] However, they may do even better when psychological treatment is added in as well, and medication should only be used in serious cases.[18]

To sum up, there are pretty effective treatments for most of the common mental disturbances of childhood. But when it comes to psychological treatments, there are four key points to be made. The first is the importance of the training of the therapist. For example, in one particular trial of parent training for antisocial behavior, the therapists were independently rated for their skill before the study began. In the study the top third of therapists were then found to improve the social behavior of the children by more than one standard deviation. As figure 13.1 shows, the least effective therapists actually had a negative effect— which bad therapy can indeed always have. This shows the huge importance of a professionally trained workforce.

Next, the treatment has bigger effects the bigger the problem (provided the problem is not overwhelming). This reinforces the importance of diagnosis and good assessment. As in all therapy, there is some fading of effects, and there are strong arguments for a "dental care" model where children (in this case) are seen again at intervals once the main treatment is over, for booster sessions. And finally, many treatments that sound perfectly plausible make no difference. For example, sending badly behaved children to summer

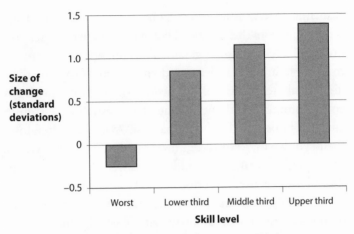

Figure 13.1. Impact of therapist skill on children's anti-social behavior.

camps with other similar children makes them no less criminal, nor do harsh boot camps.[19] Both are based on a faulty understanding of human nature. But, as we have seen, other treatments based on better models of human nature can also fail if they are not sufficiently structured.

IAPT for the Young

In 2010 the British government decided to ensure that children received treatment for which there was strong evidence of effectiveness. This involved a radical reform of mental health services for children. The situation for children was different from that for adults, where in much of the country there was virtually no psychological therapy available at all for depression or anxiety. For children, by contrast, there were already psychologically based services available throughout the country, employing nearly 10,000 people. But they were hard to access unless the child was extremely disturbed. And surveys showed that much of the treatment they provided was not based on any evidence of effectiveness. In a 2008 survey less than half the services said they were implementing NICE guidelines. In another survey half the therapists said they used CBT for less than one-fifth of their cases, and two-thirds felt they needed more training in child-focused CBT.[20]

So the government launched a four-year program to upgrade the service. This Children and Young People's IAPT program has the same two elements as for adults: a training program (focused on CBT, parent training, systemic family therapy, and interpersonal therapy) and a program for developing better services. Every service included in the program has to monitor the children's progress on a session-by-session basis, which provides the therapist with accurate knowledge about how the child is doing and enables the therapist's supervisor to focus on ways of achieving more successful outcomes.

There is a long way to go, especially when reduced government funding of local authorities recently led to devastating cuts in child mental health services But, despite this, there is already a huge new sense of energy in these services. By the end of this decade, Britain will be offering first-class NICE-recommended treatment to very many more of its troubled children. This will give them enormously improved chances of living happier, healthier, and more productive lives. It will be a huge achievement.

But there is another huge issue—of access. At the moment in Britain, as in most countries, a child has to be quite severely troubled to be seen by any specialist service.

Children with mild to moderate problems, which seriously affect their learning and their friendships, are rarely seen. This needs to change. Each school should have a named part-time therapist available to see children in the school. There should be a target of seeing at least 33% of need by 2020. This will mean a major expansion of provision by at least a quarter by 2020.

Children in distress need other support too. They need teachers—who will understand and who in most cases are best placed (after parents) to spot their distress. And, if things are bad enough, the children will also need help from social workers, the police, and the courts. Close collaboration between all these is essential, but therapy must be part of it.

It is hugely unjust that so many children worldwide are denied help with their mental health.[21] They cannot argue the case for themselves, and their parents are often inhibited by a sense of shame. But whole societies are thereby the poorer. We need a completely new priority for treating our troubled children.

It would be even better if we could prevent them becoming troubled in the first place. But how?

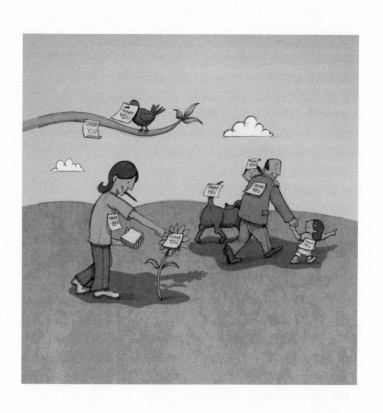

14 * Can We Prevent Mental Illness?

> I am the master of my fate:
> I am the captain of my soul.
>
> *William Ernest Henley, "Invictus"*

In 1977 David Olds launched his first trial of "Nurse-Family Partnerships" in the Appalachian region of New York State. The aim was to improve the way in which poor, teenage, first-time mothers bring up their children. Trained nurses visited nearly two hundred mothers roughly once a month during pregnancy and for the following two years. Having gained the trust of the mother, the nurse had structured ("manualized") conversations with her about three main sets of issues: healthy living for mother and child, the emotional care of the child, and the mother's own ambitions for what sort of person she wanted to be.

The children of these mothers have now been followed up for nineteen years and compared with a randomized control group. The differences in life-course are striking. Children who went through the program did better at school academically and behaved better. After leaving school, they committed much less crime. So the program was a great success both academically and in terms of reducing conduct disorder. In terms of social cost-benefit analysis, the returns from the program in terms of higher earnings and lower costs of crime gave a more than adequate yield on the initial cost of $9,600 per child.[1] The program is now being widely rolled out in Britain, with a planned enrolment of 15,000 mothers.

So people's lives can be changed for the better through the right kind of help. But how in general can we prevent mental illness and promote well-being? There are two main ways. One is through a better, more civilized and more mental health conscious society, as we will discuss in the next chapter. But can we not earlier on, while people are still children, inoculate them with the capacity to resist mental illness throughout their lives?

We are beginning to know how to.[2] The science is much less developed than it is in treating illness once it arises. Few preventive studies have long follow-ups, and many programs that look quite sensible make little difference—often because they are far too short.[3]

Early Interventions

But to build confidence, let us begin with three interventions that have, like Nurse-Family Partnerships, documented major lasting effects upon behavior. The first is the well-known Perry Pre-School project in the US state of Michigan. This was a randomized controlled trial for high-risk African American children ages three and four. They spent two years in school for half the day, and the mothers were also visited at home each week. Thereafter, the children from the program did much better academically and behaved better than the controls, while as adults they were half as likely to be arrested for criminal conduct than those in the control group. When all the benefits and costs are assessed in terms of monetary value, it turned out that the real rate of return was 7–10% per annum—higher than the long-term yield on equities.[4]

Similarly good results were found from the so-called Abecedarian Project in North Carolina. This provided all-day play-based child care for deprived children from birth to the age of five.[5] By the age of twenty-one these children had done better at school, earned more, and been less involved in crime or on welfare than the randomized controls.

These were expensive programs for highly targeted groups of children. A less expensive program (per head) was aimed at all the children in a group of schools in deprived areas of Baltimore. In the Good Behavior Game, each primary school first-year class is divided into three teams and each team is scored according to the number of times a member of the team breaks one of the behavior rules. If there are fewer than five infringements, *all* members of the team get a reward. Children in the treatment and control groups were followed right up to the ages of nineteen to twenty-one, and those in the treatment group had significantly lower use of drugs, alcohol, and tobacco, and significantly lower frequency of antisocial personality disorder.[6]

However, one should always be careful about generalizing from individual experiments, since once in a while an intervention will by chance appear effective even if it is not.[7] To overcome this problem we need a meta-analysis that summarizes the results of a number of experiments.[8] For children of school age, there have now been enough experiments to make this possible.

Social and Emotional Learning

From a mental health point of view, the main aim must be that children can understand and manage their own

Table 14.1. Programs of social and emotional learning have good effects

	Average gain (in percentile points)	(Number of programs)
Effect on		
Emotional well-being	9	(106)
Conduct	9	(112)
Academic performance	11	(35)

emotions—and understand and empathize with the feelings of others. Learning to do this involves both social and emotional learning (SEL).

CASEL, or the Collaborative for Academic, Social, and Emotional Learning, is a consortium of people interested in promoting the spread of social and emotional learning in the United States. It has a variety of distinguished patrons and has recently conducted an impressive meta-analysis of school-based SEL programs that are "universal"—that is, aimed at the whole range of children. Half of the programs were for primary-age children and half for middle or upper secondary-age children. The results were encouraging. The average program had significant immediate effects on emotional well-being, conduct, and academic performance. These effects are given in table 14.1. As it shows, the children who took these programs increased their emotional well-being and behavior by 9 points (in a ranking of children from 1 to 100). But, strikingly, their schoolwork also improved by at least as much.[9]

Isn't it obvious that happier children learn better? You would think so, but in Britain we have influential politicians who think that social and emotional learning is a distraction from the proper role of schools, which is to focus on academic performance. The evidence, however, speaks for itself: the two objectives are not alternatives; they reinforce each other.

So the first lesson that emerges is that *programs aimed at emotional well-being are also good for academic achievement.* A second lesson is that *most programs benefit children with problems more than they benefit children with fewer problems.*[10] This might seem like an argument for greater targeting, but that is not necessarily so. For one thing, targeting involves singling out children at risk, which may itself be harmful; and, second, universal programs help to create a climate of psychological awareness from which those in need benefit most.

A third key finding of the CASEL analysis is that programs work best if they are well structured with a clear, explicit sequence and require active participation by the students. In fact *the best programs are "manualized"*—there is a manual that gives detailed guidance to the teacher. It is easy to see how important this is from Britain's recent experience with its national program called SEAL—Social and Emotional Aspects of Learning. This is based on the same ideas as CBT and encapsulated in the phrases "emotional intelligence" and "social intelligence."[11] But the program goes no further than issuing lists of topics and possible materials; it has no structured procedure. When evaluators compared the SEAL program in secondary schools with a control group, they found that "it failed to impact significantly upon pupils' social and emotional skills, general mental health difficulties, pro-social behavior or behavior problems."[12] It needed to be much more manualized. This is not a device to deskill the teacher, any more than protocols for surgery deskill the surgeon. It is the best guarantee of quality and effectiveness.

A fourth finding is that *programs about what not to do are rarely successful.* This is true whether they are about sex, drugs, alcohol, tobacco, or crime.[13] For example, in the original Scared Straight program in the United States, young people were taken into prison to see how horrible it is. Twenty years later the kids who participated said the program had helped them keep out of trouble. But the research showed that, compared with the control group, more of them had broken the law. Similar results were found in all seven of the other "scared straight" projects that have been evaluated. Similarly, to discourage drugs and alcohol the DARE program pays for police officers to go into schools to explain the dangers involved. The result? More drinking and drug taking than in the control group. And yet the program is used in 75% of US school districts.

These are classic examples of apparently sensible treatments—like posttrauma psychological debriefing—which actually make things worse. There are others that simply have no effect—like paying teenage mothers to have no more babies. What do work are programs that focus on positive living—Do's rather than Don'ts. As a simple example, teenage mothers who are offered opportunities for volunteering have fewer babies. So the test of a good program is that it focuses on the positive and that it is manualized, so that it does not depend for success on an outstanding teacher.

Another quite general finding about programs is that *their effects fade over time.*[14] And a final finding is that their initial effects are on average quite small—a typical program raises the average person's well-being six months after the end of the program by approaching 0.25 standard deviations—or an increase of 10 percentile points. And that effect then fades.

The conclusion is that *these programs are far too small—* many of them lasting not more than twenty hours. As Aristotle always stressed, the key to a good character is good habits.[15] These are only acquired through continual repetition. Can we really expect a twenty-hour program to change many children's lives? It doesn't seem reasonable to do so.[16] We are still in the very early days of the psychological revolution, where little toeholds like twenty hours feel like real progress. But what we really need is for the development of social and emotional skills to become a key objective for all schools, secondary as well as primary.

An Experiment

The approach to this should be based on evidence, not on inspired guesswork. First there has to be a radical change in the whole ethos of the school.[17] At the same time children would benefit from a complete SEL curriculum for at least one hour a week throughout their school life, based on manualized programs that have been tested and found to be effective. We have searched the world for school-based programs that have been shown to have good effects on mental well-being; on responsible social and sexual relationships; and on consumption of alcohol, tobacco, and drugs. From the best of these we have designed a weekly curriculum for eleven- to fourteen-year-olds and are testing it in thirty schools.[18] The curriculum will cover not only social and emotional learning but also sex and relationships, parenting, healthy living, mental health, media awareness and mindfulness.[19] We shall see how it does.

Resilience

It may be worth discussing two features of our experiment in more detail. The first is resilience. Our proposed curriculum starts with the Penn Resilience Program, which was produced under the leadership of Martin Seligman. Seligman was one of Aaron Beck's early disciples, and he has gone on to apply the ideas of CBT to the enhancement of well-being rather than just the reduction of ill-being. For this purpose he has developed what he calls Positive Psychology, which is now a worldwide movement.[20] His resilience program takes eighteen hours, with the children in groups of fifteen. Teachers get ten days' training. In a meta-analysis the average effect of the program has been similar to those in the CASEL analysis quoted earlier, and it is also subject to fading—except that in a British trial the academic effect (5 percentile points) persisted over the following two years.[21]

The Resilience Program is now being used for every soldier in the US Army, with the aim of reducing the incidence of posttraumatic stress disorder after traumatic experiences on the battlefield.[22] General Casey is the five-star general who commissioned this, and his impressive objective is that "every soldier should be as psychologically fit as he is physically fit." The first head of this training program in the army was Brigadier General Cornum, who became world famous when she was captured in the first Gulf War and molested and tortured by Iraqi troops. If she doesn't know about resilience, who does?

Mindfulness

A second key feature of our experiment will be mindfulness. This will be an integral part of every class. Mindfulness is one of the oldest forms of psychological practice, developed by the Buddha or even earlier and still used all over the world. During mindfulness training you learn to focus your attention on what is happening in the present moment, in a spirit of nonjudgmental acceptance. You begin by focusing on your own body, especially your breathing, simply observing your sensations with friendly curiosity. You then observe your thoughts and emotions, and how they come and go.

You notice that there are two stages in bad feeling—first there is some external trigger and then there is the way the mind makes things worse by the way it reacts. You learn not to react in an aversive way pushing away bad experience, but rather in a friendly, approaching manner. You observe yourself, as it were, from outside so that you cease to be the prisoner of your thoughts and feelings.[23] This trains you in self-compassion, and through that in compassion for others.

By now millions of people in the West have taken the Mindfulness-Based Stress Reduction (MBSR) course developed by Jon Kabat-Zinn at the University of Massachusetts. The standard course is a weekly session for eight weeks, but the real work is the daily period of practice, which aims to set a pattern for the rest of your life. The course has been

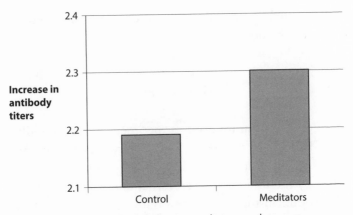

Figure 14.1. When injected with flu vaccine, meditators produce more antibodies.

subjected to rigorous evaluation, especially among groups of adults.[24] It improves mood and sleep, reduces substance abuse, improves concentration, and increases empathy.[25] Correspondingly, it increases the gray matter in the brain areas critical for learning and the regulation of emotion.[26]

Mindfulness is also good for your physical health. Just as stress disturbs the production of cortisol (the "fight or flight" hormone) and weakens the immune system, so MBSR improves these. In one study, people were given flu injections four months after the course was over.[27] As figure 14.1 shows, people who had taken this course produced far more antibodies than the control group.

It is perhaps not surprising that all US marines are now given mindfulness training. This training has also been found to work well with children and young people.[28] There have been fewer trials with them than with adults, but the results are similar. Their mental health improves and so does their behavior.

This is bound to improve learning.[29] So there is much to be said for a short practice of mindfulness, such as the three-minute "breathing space," as the prelude to every lesson. This can also contribute mightily to the problem of indiscipline in schools, which blights the life of so many young people.

Behavior at School

Bad behavior in school is a taboo subject. It's not politically correct to talk about it and, shockingly, there are no good time series that show whether it is getting worse or better.[30] The politically correct view is that if you have a good lesson plan there will be no disorder. But for many children and their parents, disorder in their schools is a major issue. In a US national sample of twelve- to eighteen-year-olds, only 29% said their school provided a caring, encouraging environment.[31] In a survey of children ages eleven and fourteen in Britain's metropolitan areas, 29% said that every day other pupils tried to disrupt their lessons, and 43% said that other pupils were "always" or "often" so noisy they found it difficult to work.[32]

Teachers say the same. In a representative survey, teachers reported that in their "daily experience" 43% experienced disruption in their lessons; 47% experienced answering back; 19% experienced persistent and malicious disruptive behavior, including open defiance; 16% experienced a pupil threatening violence to another pupil; and 9% experienced damage to property. They also reported that at least "on a weekly basis" 7% themselves experienced pushing/touching or other unwanted physical contact, 6% witnessed violence by a pupil to another member of staff, and 2% experienced threats of violence to teachers from parents.[33]

Most of these problems would disappear if there were better order in the classroom. This is a skill that can be systematically taught in an evidence-based way. The course takes around three to five days in college, with occasional follow-ups. Teachers are taught the same basic skills as are taught to parents in the Incredible Years parent training. These are: (1) keep calm; (2) give as much praise as possible; and (3) give small, immediate punishments.[34] Randomized trials show how effective this training can be;[35] there are some basic principles that apply at every age and in every context.

Conclusions

There is a huge amount that professionals can do to improve the mental health of our children. At the preschool stage they can support disadvantaged parents, through programs like America's Head Start and England's Sure Start[36]—but better structured. There can also be systems whereby nurses mentor mothers at risk and health visitors screen and treat maternal depression.[37]

Once children are in school, the whole environment needs to be devoted to their well-being and not just to their academic development. As we saw in chapter 5, children's emotional development has more effect on their later well-being than their intellectual development does. Schools need to care about both, as many already do. This requires the right school ethos, but also dedicated teaching of life skills conducive to mental health. At present some 60% of US schools teach these, as do most British schools.[38] But increasingly this can be done on the basis of scientific evidence.

Life skills are some of the most difficult topics to teach. As one thirteen-year-old girl said to an English schools inspector: "I think life skills lessons should be taught by a teacher in that field, rather than a teacher who doesn't know anything about the subject but still tries to teach it to people."[39] If we had specialist teaching, this would draw into schools more psychologically minded teachers, who could act as missionaries for the caring society we discuss in the next chapter.

Schools could also measure the well-being of every child when they enter and when they leave the school. This would help them to screen for mental illness they might not otherwise notice—especially for emotional disturbance, which is less obvious than disturbed conduct. But it would also shift the goals of the school, to give greater weight to the well-being of the children.

Some do already give great weight to well-being, but they are not always thanked for it. One elementary school head teacher wrote to us of an experience he had when his school was visited by the school inspectorate:

> At the end of the week the Lead Inspector said to me, "You've got happy children, happy staff and happy parents . . ." I waited for the glowing compliment, but he went on to say, ". . . I put it to you, something is wrong." Since then our children have been subjected to an extreme regime of testing which has demoralized teachers, alienated children (especially boys) and confused parents. Good luck with your efforts—let our children have a childhood and be "educated"!!

Amen. Most schools want children to enjoy their lives and to flourish as rounded human beings. The new psychological knowledge can help in this—and it will also improve academic performance. There is a huge role for digital resources in this whole effort, provided free worldwide to health care workers, teachers, parents, and young people. This could be a major role for some enlightened donor like the Gates Foundation.[40]

But health systems and schools do not operate in a vacuum. So how can we also build a better society?

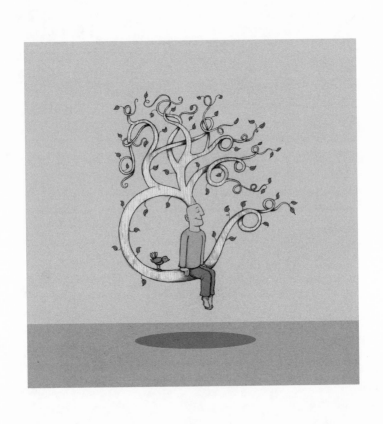

15 * Would a Better Culture Help?

> Gee, Officer Krupke, we're down on our knees,
> 'Cause no one wants a fella with a social disease.
>
> *Stephen Sondheim,* West Side Story

Is mental illness after all a social disease? Partly it is. As we saw in chapter 7, mental illness does seem to be more common in countries where there are low levels of support, trust, and cooperation, and excessive levels of competition for position.

Such competition may make us richer, but if what people actually want is a better position on the status ladder, the competition is self-defeating for society as a whole. If one person improves his place, that is necessarily at the expense of someone else who, relatively, moves down. However hard people try, there can be no overall improvement. But there is a massive cost in terms of stress and loneliness. This may be one of the many reasons why the levels of happiness and misery have not improved over the last sixty years in the United States.[1]

The conclusion is not, of course, that people should not strive. Striving is good for people, providing the goal is realistic. But much depression comes from striving for unrealistic goals. Moreover, viewed from the point of view of society, we are all affected by the goals other people pursue. Levels of trust matter, and in the United States and Britain the proportion of people who trust other people has nearly halved over the last forty years.[2]

What Goal?

What kinds of goals should our culture encourage?[3] That depends on what social outcomes we most want to see. In our view, the best outcome for any society is where there is the most happiness and above all the least misery.[4] That was the ideal proposed by the great thinkers of the eighteenth-century Enlightenment, and it remains the most convincing description of the good society. So how can we get nearer to that state?

Quite obviously, it needs every individual to contribute to that outcome. In other words, we would each adopt as our aim in life to create as much happiness as we can in the world around us and (especially) as little misery. It is a pretty demanding goal. Although our own happiness does matter, it matters no more than the happiness of all those others whom we touch. On the other hand, we are also happier if we feel committed to something bigger than our own little selves. As the Buddhist sage Shantideva said, "The person who seeks his own happiness becomes unhappy, while the happy person pursues the happiness of others."

There is a selfish side in every one of us, but there is also an altruistic side. Some of us are more altruistic than others, but it is a major role of culture to inspire and develop our altruistic side. As W. H. Auden said, "We must love one another or die."

So how can we promote a more humane society? Every organization has a role to play: families, schools, business, media, governments, and spiritual movements. As we saw in chapter 7, they all matter.

Parents

Parents are of course crucial. Their love of a child is vital for the child's self-love, and the relationship between the parents is the child's first role model of how human beings relate to each other. Some parents are worse than others at loving their children, and some are not as good at loving each other. But there is plenty we can do if we want to improve the quality of parenting.

First, we can include it in school as part of the teaching of life skills. We can teach adolescents the awesome responsibility of becoming a parent and also the emotional issues involved in relating to their future children and to the children's other parent.[5] Second, when parents produce their first child we can offer both of them classes, not only on physical childbirth and child care, but also on the emotional issues involved—how to relate to the child and how to stop the child dividing the parents (as so often happens).[6] Ideally these classes would be free—just think how much they could improve the quality of our lives.

But what happens if the parents begin to fall out? Society has a huge interest in reducing conflict within families. Early help is essential, and it would make a huge difference if the couples' therapy we described earlier were readily available. The ideal is to restore the bond between the parents—an amicable separation is often the second best.

How, more generally, can we increase the stability of family life? It must largely depend on the values people bring to their relationships. If people were even a little bit more altruistic, it would make a real difference. But there is also the issue of priorities—who comes first in the claims on our altruism? Because family life is so important, for many people it is going to be the family. And who within the family? Many parents greatly underestimate how much children care about how their parents get along with each other. In a British survey, teenagers and parents were asked whether they agreed with the statement: "Parents getting on well is one of the most important factors in raising happy children." Seven in ten of the teenagers agreed, but only a third of the parents did so.[7]

How can we improve our relationship with our partners? A natural way to think is, "I must act so that my partner loves me more." That is not an altruistic motivation. It is less likely to work than the following resolution: "I must give top priority to maintaining my own love for my partner." That has a real chance.

Schools

Next in a child's life comes school. Schools have us in their hands at the most formative time of our lives. As Aristotle saw, people behave well if that has become their habit, and it is a habit that can be learned. But unfortunately schools in the West have increasingly become exam factories. They need to build character as well as competence.

One element in this can be the life skills training we have already discussed. But another is the ethos of values that permeates the whole life of the school. An obvious number-one value is respect—in the way teachers behave to each other and to the children, and in the way the children and the parents behave. But respect goes only so far—what also matters is concern. Morality goes beyond what you "don't" do. Suppose children grew up with the goal in life of creating as much happiness in the world around them as possible, and as little misery. Different schools would find different languages to express this ideal. But each would find its own way of breeding idealism. We will not get a decent society if teachers ceaselessly appeal to the selfish instincts of their children—like their wish to beat others in exams or to earn lots of money when they leave school. Children need to have noble role models, and teachers need to feel totally comfortable when talking about their own values, rather than just saying to the children, "What do you think?"

Business

If we turn to the world of work, employers can make a world of difference to their workers. Nine hundred working women in Texas were asked to reconstruct the previous day and to record for each episode what they were doing, how they felt, and who they were with.[8] Their worst time of day was when they were with their line manager. This says something pretty bad about the quality of line management. In a recent report for the World Economic Forum, one key recommendation was that line managers be appointed on the basis of their ability to lead and inspire, and not simply for their technical competence.[9]

But what principles of work organization lead to contented workers, and are these principles good for profits? Research reveals three basic principles.[10] First, it helps if workers are given clear, feasible goals, and a clear understanding of how they fit into a picture that is bigger than just them. Second, it helps if they are given the greatest possible freedom in how they achieve their goals. And third, it helps if they have regular support and feedback on how they are doing. Such workplaces would generate workers who are not only "engaged" (which employers always want) but also enjoying their work. Employers would also avoid forms of incentive pay that generate excessive pressure.[11]

There is in fact good evidence that happy workplaces are also more productive. Much of the evidence is of the post hoc, ergo propter hoc variety, without a control group. A management consultant goes into a firm, conducts a survey of job satisfaction, and then helps the firm reorganize the less happy departments. In the years that follow productivity rises.[12]

Possibly more impressive is an interesting comparative analysis of rates of return on shareholders' equity.[13] The analysis focuses on one hundred US companies that (based on employee surveys) were judged to be the "100 Best Places to Work" in 1985. The share prices of those companies were followed for the next twenty-five years and compared with the share prices of all other US listed companies. After twenty-five years, money invested in the 100 Best Places to Work was worth 50% more than the same amount of money invested in other companies.

How, specifically, would a good company handle the mental health problems of its workers? These may arise from issues at the workplace, but in over three-quarters of cases the main problem lies elsewhere (in the family or simply in the individual). But how the company reacts can be crucial, and every firm needs a code of practice for handling these problems. First, line managers would be aware that these problems are quite common, and if they thought a colleague had a problem, they would ask about it. Second, if a person goes absent, their line manager would (in a caring way) ask what the problem is. It would be the line manager not the Human Resources Department who did this, since the line manager ought to care most and is best placed to organize any work adjustment that is needed. Third, if there were a mental health problem, people would be offered treatment either within the firm's occupational health service (on a confidential basis) or through the worker's standard health care system. There would also be standard ways of easing a person's return to work (via fewer hours or less responsibility, as needed). And finally, the company may offer preventive courses in stress management, such as the Mindfulness-Based Stress Reduction program, to help prevent the problem in the first place.

What of the firm's responsibilities to its consumers? An ethical company does not sell things it does not consider good for people. Unfortunately many banks, drug companies, insurance companies, and others have done just this, and made a lot of money doing it.

Media and Advertising

The same is true of the media. In one recent survey it was found that only 16% of the content of the average British newspaper is positive.[14] This has the very peculiar result that when people are asked what the world is like in general, they always give a more dismal report than they give of their own experience.

If we ask why the media give such a biased picture, it is because good news does not sell as well as bad news. This may reflect the negative side of human nature, which can get short-run pleasure from the discomfort or shortcomings of others. No one would advocate censorship on that account. But responsible journalism should include the aim of celebrating what is good. One British newspaper now runs a third leader column titled "In praise of . . ."

Press freedom is precious, but we can still criticize the media if they lie or if they deliberately appeal to our worst natures. We need journalism to be a proper profession with a code of conduct and disciplinary procedures for those who break it.[15]

Advertising poses particular problems. While the company that advertises is only trying to sell more of a specific product, the advertising industry as a whole makes us want more than we otherwise would—and thus makes us less contented with what we have. So we would benefit from less advertising. This means there is a good case for extra taxes on advertising.[16] Since alcohol is such a problem, the advertising of it could well be banned.[17]

Government

That brings us to the role of government. As Thomas Jefferson said, "The care of human life and happiness . . . is the . . . only legitimate object of good government."[18] We agree. It is difficult to think of any other reason for government activity. Governments exist to promote happiness, and especially (we would add) to reduce misery.[19]

This perspective has enormous implications. It means that governments would judge their success not by the growth of national income but by the elimination of misery and the growth of happiness. For this reason more and more countries are taking regular official measurements of the happiness of their peoples. The lead has come from the club of rich nations, the OECD, which had its first conference on "What Is Progress?" in 2004. The first countries to officially measure the happiness of the nation were Britain and Bhutan, but now nearly all OECD countries are doing it in a standard way.[20]

The next step, after measuring happiness, is to try to increase it. That requires a deep quantitative understanding of what causes happiness and by how much. That should now become one of the principal aims of social science research. We already know that it will involve a radical change of priorities for all our countries. We know that the main external factor affecting a person's happiness is not income but the quality of a person's relationships (in the family, through work, and in the community). And the main internal factor is mental health, followed by physical health.[21] This means that to increase happiness we have to devote more resources to mental health above all, but also to physical health, child support, family support, old age support, and job training.

At the margin, money for these purposes would do more to increase happiness than leaving the money for families to spend on other things. This is not a matter of ideology, and it has nothing to do with more or less equality. It is a simple consequence of the evidence. For example, in an important study of British children ages ten to fifteen, it was found that family income per head had no effect on whether the children were happy about their lives. What mattered most was the quality of their human relationships—whether their parents were still together, whether the other children at school behaved in class, whether they played a sport.[22]

This suggests we need more government expenditure on supporting family relationships and social activity, and relatively less focus on pure money income.[23]

Again, if well-being rather than income is the goal, this has profound consequences for the management of the economy. According to the Chicago school of economics we should be willing to tolerate a sequence of recessions and booms if this leads to faster overall growth in incomes.[24] Swayed by this philosophy, politicians deregulated the banks when they promised faster growth. But the cost was a huge recession and mass unemployment, causing major unhappiness, family tensions, and mental breakdown. Instead, the government should always give overriding importance to economic stability.[25]

And what, finally, of inequality? First, there is a simple point about the value of extra money to different people. Extra money makes more difference to a poor person than to a rich one. To be precise, an extra dollar to a poor person will give him ten times more extra happiness than that extra dollar would give to another person who is already ten times richer.[26] This has always been the main argument for redistributing income.

But inequality seems to have a wider impact on happiness than can be explained by this fact. We can begin with the much-publicized results in Richard Wilkinson and Kate Pickett's book, *The Spirit Level*. Comparing across countries and across US states, they find that income inequality is correlated with lower well-being of many kinds.[27] But strikingly they find that inequality is bad for the rich as well as for the poor. For example, rich people in Sweden are healthier than rich people in Britain, even though the rich people in Sweden are poorer than the rich people in

Britain. For this to happen, inequality must be working not just through its effect on individual purchasing power but also through the whole ethos of society.

The Spirit Level is only one of many studies on this issue, including some that also allow for other possible factors as well as income inequality.[28] Not all these studies find that income inequality matters. What is more certain is that the ethos of a society matters deeply. An egalitarian ethos may work through many channels, making it difficult to isolate the effect of each individual channel. But how can we influence the ethos itself?

Spiritual Movements

Ultimately, the culture of a society depends on what individuals believe. Countless influences channel these beliefs—above all, schools and the media. But further back in the chain come the originators of the ideas, most commonly writers, academics, preachers, and artists. We should never overlook the power of such people and the movements they engender.

An interesting example comes from the cultural changes in Britain between 1789 and 1834. Before 1789 anyone who talked about the reformation of society was accused of "cant," and there was little worse that you could be accused of.[29] It was a period of easy sex, much drunkenness, and harsh ill treatment of children, animals, "lunatics," prisoners, and slaves. By 1834 all talk of cant had gone, slavery had been abolished, and a wave of social reform was under way. Behind all this were the powerful ideas of evangelicalism and the philosophy of the Enlightenment.

What idea is there now that can change our present culture and make it more caring? Why not the philosophy of the well-being movement, which is now a worldwide phenomenon? This proposes a new goal for a society (greater happiness and less misery) plus the means to achieve it (more altruism and more attention to the inner life). It offers both a philosophy and scientific evidence on how we can do better. The strongest science derives from CBT, and from Positive Psychology, which applies the ideas of CBT to the lives of everybody.[30] This is strongly complemented by the wisdom of the East, where the Buddhist practice of mindfulness takes many people further than they can reach through Positive Psychology alone: the number of people who meditate is growing rapidly.[31]

This well-being revolution has been building up for many years, but it has few institutional forms to carry it forward. That was the reason for founding Action for Happiness. This is a movement founded in 2011 and based on the principles outlined in this chapter. Its members pledge to try to create more happiness in the world and less misery. Their website gives the members access to the treasures of Positive Psychology and to other suggested ways of raising happiness for yourself and for others.[32] But to live well is not easy, and there is strength in numbers. So increasingly the movement's 250,000 online followers from over one hundred countries are forming groups to support one another in living well. The movement now provides a course of eight sessions called "Exploring What Matters," where groups of people gather together to discuss their goals in life. When the course is over, the group continues to meet and support one another's beliefs, in the same way that faith organizations worldwide have done for centuries.

Faith organizations are still of course the main spiritual organizations in today's world. They do good works for others and provide comfort and support to their members.[33] Even if many people cannot accept their creeds, they are key allies in any movement to ensure that we give proper weight to the inner life.

Like faith organizations, the well-being movement is independent of Left or Right. It calls for a new concept of deprivation, where you are deprived if you cannot enjoy your life—whether or not that is due to lack of money. To recognize this kind of deprivation, and to prevent it, requires a major change in our culture and major improvements in how we act in schools, in families, and in business.

When the chief executive of Action for Happiness was being appointed, one of the candidates for the job reported that he had searched the web for other organizations whose title included the word "happiness." This was the reply on his screen: "Your search for happiness has yielded no results."

We can do better than that, especially if we give proper attention to mental health. And, even if you disagree with some of this chapter, you can still agree with everything else we say about the importance of mental health. Apart perhaps from global warming, there is no other major problem that is so neglected worldwide.

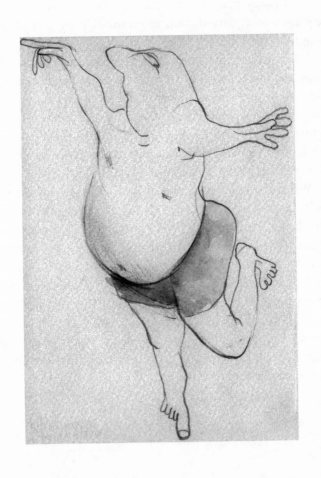

16 * Stop This Pain

Dear Lord Layard,

My husband was referred for CBT in April last year. Four
months later he had a telephone assessment and was put
on a waiting list. Five months after that his mental health
really deteriorated. We begged for help because we were
frightened of him losing his job and us our home. Three
months later that happened.

This is typical of letters we receive each week. Worldwide
there are hundreds of millions of people whose situation
is equally desperate. It is difficult to excuse this. For as this
book shows, common mental illness is not only the biggest
source of misery in our countries; it is also the source of
misery we can most easily address. Here are the key facts:

- Depression and anxiety account for more of the misery in
  Western societies than physical illness does. And they account for very much more misery than is due to poverty
  or unemployment. So the front line in the fight against
  misery is the fight against mental illness.
- Really effective remedies exist. Psychological therapies
  taking less than sixteen sessions produce 50% recovery
  rates that are often permanent, and, when they are not,
  they greatly reduce the risk of relapse.
- These life-changing therapies are not expensive to the
  health care system. Their gross cost per patient is less than
  the cost of six months' treatment for diabetes.[1] Moreover,
  this cost is mostly recouped in the reduced cost of physical health care for people who have physical as well as

mental health problems. On top of that there is the saving on welfare payments. So there would be no net cost in making these therapies more widely available.

- Yet, while over 90% of diabetes sufferers receive treatment for their condition, under a third of adults with diagnosable mental illness do so. This is largely because good evidence-based psychological therapy is not readily available.
- The same is true of children. Good treatments exist but only a quarter of those who need help are in treatment. Yet over half of all children who are mentally ill also become mentally ill as adults.
- This undertreatment is a gross injustice. It is sheer discrimination against those who are mentally ill, and an abuse of human rights.
- It is also a gross inefficiency. For mental illness imposes huge costs on the rest of society. It causes family break-up, crime, substance abuse, welfare dependence, and massive needs for physical health care.

It is high time for a quite new approach. We need to implement one very simple principle: *evidence-based treatment should be as available for mental as for physical illness*. If implemented everywhere, that would be a worldwide revolution. It would probably do more to make the world a happier place than any other way of spending the same amount of money.

Parity of Esteem

On October 12, 1984, the British Cabinet members were staying with their spouses in the Grand Hotel in Brighton for the Conservative Party conference. Just before 3:00 a.m. there was a massive explosion as Irish Republicans unleashed a bomb that destroyed great parts of the building. One of the victims was Margaret Tebbit, wife of then Secretary of State for Trade. Most of her body was paralyzed for life. Yet earlier in her life she had experienced postnatal depression and she insists that that was worse than her paralysis.[2]

Health services take immense trouble over physical paralysis, but most postnatal depression remains untreated. Everywhere in the world there is massive discrimination against the millions in despair or torment due to mental illness. Yet a number of countries, including the United States and Britain, have now passed laws establishing parity of esteem for mental and physical health.[3]

What in practice should parity of esteem mean?

- First, cost-effective psychological therapy for those who want it would become as available as medication. In England doctors who prescribe medication often do so contrary to the NICE guidelines because there are no psychological therapy services to which they can refer their patients. Adequate psychological therapy services would be able to treat at least 4% of the adult population each year—that is a quarter of those with diagnosable depression or anxiety disorders.
- Access to therapy would be rapid, with waiting times similar to those for urgent physical care. Most patients should be treated by a therapist within a month of referral. The therapy would be evidence-based, but it would not be the cheapest possible variant that funders could get away with—like "six sessions maximum." We would never propose half a course of treatment for a physical

condition, nor should we for a mental illness. We should provide what all readers of this book would want to receive if they needed it.

- All therapy would be provided in a structured way, where the therapists are measuring outcomes on a session-by-session basis, and getting regular supervision on their cases. Normally this is best organized by having therapists working in a team. Outcome data would be publicly available so that it becomes obvious how well a service is doing and how it compares with the services that are doing best.

- Even the best treatments do not always work, and even when they do there is often the danger of relapse. So all services would be much more ready to provide booster sessions to people whose treatment has worked, and an alternative treatment for those where it has failed.

- The rest of the health services would be much more psychologically aware. This is particularly true of family doctors and nurses. In their training, all family doctors would do a period of training in the treatment of depression and anxiety disorders. One such experiment on the island of Gotland in Sweden showed dramatic results—with hospital admissions for depression falling for a time by 70% and suicides by a similar amount.[4]

- We are still at the very beginning of the psychological revolution. Scientific methods have only been widely applied to designing therapies for about twenty-five years. And only a limited range of therapies has been at all fully developed. There is currently far too little money for research on mental illness. In Britain it gets only 5% of the health research budget, although it accounts for 23% of the "burden of disease." This must change. Proper psychological trials are expensive, and research money is needed to cover the design and implementation of better therapies as well as their evaluation. More work is also needed on the biological element in mental illness, and on the scope for better biological treatments. So far much of this work has been left to the drug companies, but progress is difficult and the drug companies are losing interest. We need a major advance in the basic biological science, and this needs public funding.

- Health service provision would no longer be made on the basis of who shouts loudest—which often means the big drug companies and those who want their products. Health service planning would start with an analysis of the burden of disease and the cost effectiveness of available treatments.[5] Most money would then go to those problems where there is the largest need and to those treatments that are the most cost effective. On both criteria mental health would be a top priority.

Prevention

The top need is for parity of treatment when people are ill. But we should also do all we can to prevent mental illness before it occurs. The last two chapters were about this. But what are the chances of success?

They are good. Already our societies are becoming more psychologically literate. Nine out of ten people believe it is "more acceptable to talk about emotional problems than it was in the past."[6] But there is a long way to go in reducing the stigma of mental illness and increasing our emotional literacy. Crystal gazing, here are a few outrageous suggestions about where our countries might be in twenty-five years' time.

First, all schools will have the emotional well-being of their children as an important, explicit objective. The whole school ethos will reflect this. All primary school teachers will be taught evidence-based ways of fostering emotional literacy in their children. In secondary schools the teaching of life skills will be a separate subject based on evidence, and those who teach it will be specially trained. Schools will routinely measure the well-being of their children, and all teachers will be taught to understand mental illness and how it can be helped.

Second, our society will be less macho. There will be more emphasis on collaboration and less on competition. Recent drops in crime rates in almost all developed countries may already reflect a growth in social responsibility.[7] Other evidence of this is falling teenage pregnancy and falling alcohol and drug consumption among the young. Future changes will see a continuing feminization of our values—with more importance attached to relationships and to peaceable and harmonious living. This will be helped greatly as more women come to the top of their professions. The caring professions will acquire more prestige and a greater share of national resources.

Third, there will be a massive impact of Eastern values and practices. Meditative practices of various kinds will become the dominant mode of spirituality. And mindfulness may become a regular practice taught in schools and practiced by many adults.

Fourth, in at least some countries there will be a cabinet minister for mental health. Clearly, there should be a minister for each important area of human life. If there is a cabinet minister for transport or for the environment, there should surely be one for mental health, which has such a profound impact on all our lives. For the sake of proper coordination there might continue to be one ministry of health. But if mental health is taken seriously enough, it will have to have its own cabinet minister.

A New Concept of Deprivation

Mental health is not only a part of our personal health—it is also something that affects all aspects of our lives. It affects behavior in our schools, the safety of our streets, and the functioning of our families. Most social work deals with the consequences of mental illness. We need a new concept of deprivation, where you are deprived if you cannot enjoy your life, whatever the reason.

It is mainly because we did not tackle mental health problems that the postwar vision of a happier society failed to come about. What Sir William Beveridge and politicians worldwide overlooked was the person within. We were told that material prosperity, full employment, and better physical health would solve our problems, and they did not. There remains a sixth giant to be slain: it is mental illness.

Future generations will be amazed at how blind we were. They will also be amazed that we were so cruel. When we look back at earlier generations, we are shocked by how they treated slaves, or women and children in the mines, or people with physical disabilities. Our successors will be amazed at how we treat people today who are mentally ill—how we routinely ignore their desperate pleas for psychological support.

There is only one excuse—that until recently there was little that could be done for people who are mentally ill. But there have now been great psychological discoveries, which have produced treatments for depression, anxiety, and conduct disorder more cost effective than most treatments for physical illness.

How can we get these treatments to the people who need them? Only if people are much more active in demanding that this happens. It is not reasonable to expect much activism from those who are mentally ill or their relatives: they are naturally reticent. It is all of us who should be demanding change. This should be high on the political platform of every party.

For activists in every country, this is your cause.

OUR THANKS

This book owes so much to so many. First of all are the key people who helped develop and launch the IAPT program—both for adults and children. They include psychologists and therapists Jeremy Clarke, Peter Fonagy, Stephen Pilling, David Richards, Tony Roth, and Graham Turpin; psychiatrists Louis Appleby and Stephen Scott; economist Martin Knapp; administrators James Seward, Kathryn Tyson, Kathryn Pugh, Karen Turner, Jeremy Heywood, and the national IAPT team, as well as ministers of health Alan Johnson, Andy Burnham, Andrew Lansley, Jeremy Hunt, Paul Burstow, and Norman Lamb.

Without the commitment of all these people the program would never have happened. But it would have achieved nothing without the skill, passion, and dedication of the thousands of therapists who have made it a transformational experience for hundreds of thousands of their patients.

We also want to thank all the others who have helped us understand what needed to happen. Most important have been the members of the LSE Centre for Economic Performance's Mental Health Policy Group, which produced two major reports that helped develop the arguments in the book. The first was the *Depression Report*, published in 2006, and the second, published in 2012, was called *How Mental Illness Loses Out in the NHS*. Members of the group, for one or both reports, were Sube Banerjee, Stuart Bell, Stephen Field, Martin Knapp, Molly Meacher, Christopher Naylor, Michael Parsonage, Stefan Priebe, Stephen Scott, John Strang, Graham Thornicroft, Leslie Turnberg, Simon Wessely, and Ben Wright.

In summer 2013 a group of colleagues generously assembled at Magdalen College, Oxford, to comment on the first draft of this book. They were Alastair Campbell, Will Hutton, Stephen Hyman, Martin Knapp, Michael Marmot, Peter McGuffin, Molly Meacher, Michael Parsonage, Stephen Pilling, Stephen Scott, and Leslie Turnberg. Apart from them we have had invaluable advice and comments from Paul Bebbington, Dan Chisholm, Richard Frank, Nisha Mehta, Christopher Naylor, Nigel Rogers, Robert Plomin, Michael Rutter, Bill Sadleir, Andrew Steptoe, Graham Thornicroft, Kit Welchman, and Mark Williams.

In his exploration of how to improve psychological therapies David has been privileged to work with many gifted psychotherapy researchers including Aaron T. Beck, Anke Ehlers, Melanie Fennell, Michael Gelder, Nick Grey, Ann Hackmann, Sheena Liness, Freda McManus, Jack Rachman, Paul Salkovskis, Richard Stott, John Teasdale, Emma Warnock-Parkes, Adrian Wells, and Jennifer Wild. He also benefited from time to reflect at Stanford's Center for Advanced Study in the Behavioral Sciences. Richard's interest in psychology goes back to his parents, John and Doris, both of whom were talented Jungian therapists. Since then he has been further educated in psychology through the friendship of Daniel Kahneman, Richard Davidson, Martin Seligman, and above all David.

We are also grateful to the two delightful illustrators of the book: Nick Wadley and Matthew Johnstone. Nick's cartoons (in chapters 1, 6, 7, 8, 9, 11, and 16) were specifically drawn for us, and Matthew's (in chapters 2, 3, 4, 5, 10, 12, 13, 14, and 15) have already been published in *I Had a Black Dog* and *The Alphabet of the Human Heart*.

Throughout the project, we have had superbly professional assistance in organizing the material from Harriet Ogborn, and expert research support from Chloe Booth. We are extremely grateful for financial contributions from Sushil Wadhwani, Paul Tudor Jones, Andrew Law, Henry and Sara Bedford, Rishi Khosla, Bertrand Kan, Pavel Teplukhin, The Wellcome Trust, the National Institute for Health Research, the National Institute on Aging (grant R01AG040640), and the Rosetrees Foundation. We have had a wonderful agent, Caroline Dawnay of United Agents, and, at Princeton University Press, Seth Ditchik has done a great job.

Thank you so much, everyone.

Most of all we owe to our wives, Molly and Anke. Both are distinguished experts on mental health and incredible sources of love and support. This book is for you.

RICHARD AND DAVID

SOURCES OF TABLES AND DIAGRAMS

Figure 1.1: WHO (2008). Analysis for Western Europe by Michael Parsonage.

Figure 3.1: Global Burden of Disease Study 2010 (2012). *Global burden of diseases, injuries, and risk factors study 2010.* Seattle, Institute for Health, Metrics and Evaluation.

Table 3.1: These are UK figures and mainly relate to point prevalence. For adults in 2007: McManus et al. (2009); and for children in 2004: Green et al. (2005). For adults, we assume that the primary diagnosis for common mental disorders is divided equally between depression and anxiety disorders. We have also checked that, in the survey results, common mental disorders, psychosis, personality disorder, and severe substance dependence are mainly mutually exclusive. For children, we assume strong overlap between conduct disorder, hyperkinetic disorder, and ADHD.

Figure 3.2: Twenge et al. (2010), p. 151. Minnesota Multiphasic Personality Inventory (MMPI) Depression (D) scale scores.

Figure 3.3: WHO (2008), Western Europe. Analysis by Michael Parsonage.

Figure 3.4: WHO (2008), Western Europe. Analysis by Michael Parsonage.

Figure 3.5: WHO Mortality Database http://apps.who.int/health info/statistics/mortality/whodpms/.

Table 3.2: Ayuso-Mateos et al. (2010).

Table 3.3: Based mainly on Williams (2001), Chapter 3.

Figure 4.1: McManus et al. (2009), Green et al. (2005), and Ormel et al. (2008).

Table 4.1: McManus et al. (2009); Kessler et al. (2005c); Wittchen and Jacobi (2005); Ormel et al. (2008), Table 1.

Figure 5.1: U.S. data. See Flèche and Layard (2015) and annex 5.1.

Figure 5.2: Dolan and Metcalfe (2012).

Figure 5.3: English Longitudinal Study of Ageing (ELSA). Data supplied by Professor Andrew Steptoe of University College London.

Figure 5.4: Danese et al. (2007).

Table 5.4: New Zealand data. Fergusson et al. (2005), Table 1.

Figure 5.5: Layard et al. (2013b), based on British Cohort Study.

Figure 5.6: Layard et al. (2013b).

Figure 5.7: Layard et al. (2013b).

Table 5.1: OECD (2012), Fig. 4.2.

Table 5.2: 21 countries: OECD (2012), p. 73. Britain: Layard et al. (2007), Table 4; see also Sainsbury Centre for Mental Health (2007), p. 8.

Table 5.3: UK data. ONS Survey of child mental health: Green et al. (2005). Children are classified according to parental reports of behavior.

Figure 6.1: Welch et al. (2009).

Figure 6.3: Helliwell et al. (2013), Chapter 3, Figure 5.

Figure 7.1: Plomin et al. (2013), p. 246.

Figure 7.2: Plomin et al (2013), pp. 245, 249, 251, 252, 259, 265, 290.

Figure 7.3: Plomin et al. (2013), p. 124.

Figure 7.4: Plomin et al. (2013), p. 123.

Table 7.1: Plomin et al. (2013), p. 77.

Table 7.2: British data. Singleton and Lewis (2003).

Table 7.3: British data. Singleton and Lewis (2003).

Figure 8.1: Mayou et al. (2000).

Figure 8.2: Dobson et al. (2008), Figure 2.

Figure 8.3: DeRubeis et al. (2008).

Figure 8.4: Grey et al. (2008).

Figure 8.5: Stangier et al. (2011).

Figure 9.3: D. M. Clark et al. (1994), Table 3.

Figure 9.4: Mansell et al. (2003).

Figure 9.5: D. M. Clark et al. (2006).

Figure 10.1: Fava et al. (2004).

Figure 10.2: Ehlers et al. (2014).

Figure 10.3: Kocsis et al. (2009).

Figure 11.1: Moore et al. (2007).

Table 11.1: English data. Singleton et al. (2001), p. 91. Mental illness here refers to depression and anxiety disorders. Physical complaints refer to long-standing physical complaints.

Figure 11.2: Gulliksson et al. (2011).

Figure 12.1: IAPT data.

Table 12.1: IAPT Key Performance Indicators data. "Numbers treated" are those who had at least two sessions of treatment, and ceased treatment in the period shown. The recovery rate is the number of those treated who recovered as a percentage of those treated who were "cases" when first seen. Data are for financial years (April–March).

Figure 12.3: Department of Health, 2011/12 National Survey of Investment in Adult Mental Health Services (2012).

Figure 13.1: Scott et al. (2008).

Figure 14.1: Davidson et al. (2003).

Table 14.1: Durlak et al. (2011), Table 5. The effect sizes are .23, .22, and .27 respectively.

LIST OF ANNEXES

Available at http://cep.lse.ac.uk/layard/thriveannex.pdf

NOTES

Preface

1 "Therapy Deficit," *Nature* 489 (September 27, 2012), 473–74.

Chapter 1. What's the Problem?

1 See A. E. Clark et al. (2013), figure 5, and Layard, Mayraz, and Nickell (2010), figures 6.2, 6.4, 6.5, and 6.7. The longest series are for the United States with sporadic Gallup figures for Britain in the 1950s and 1960s. For all European countries, the Eurobarometer series begin in the early 1970s.

2 Every remark in this chapter is supported by evidence in the chapters that follow.

3 See chapter 3.

4 Sullivan et al. (2013).

5 WHO (2008).

6 Frederick and Loewenstein (1999).

7 See chapter 4.

8 See chapters 8–10.

9 See Beck (2006). Many of the basic ideas of cognitive therapy were developed simultaneously by Albert Ellis, but he did not proceed to the systematic testing of outcomes as Beck and his colleagues did.

10 There is a well-known issue of how to describe people in treatment. We generally use the word "people" but sometimes

"patients" or "clients." From surveys it appears that people prefer these words to "service user"; see Simmons et al. (2010).

11 See chapter 11.
12 Issued by the National Institute for Health and Care Excellence (NICE).
13 See chapter 13.
14 Crime is of course now falling in most Western countries, but it is still much higher than in the 1950s.
15 See chapters 14 and 15.
16 See chapter 12.
17 M. A. Sieghart, "Talking Therapy Is Natural, Effective, Fast and So Cheap," *The Times*, December 7, 2006.

Chapter 2. What Is Mental Illness?

1 *Anxious Times* 79 (Autumn 2011).
2 Veale and Willson (2011).
3 Ivison (2011).
4 For the source of this figure and others in this chapter, see chapter 3. The figures aim to represent a consensus view of prevalence in the United States, Britain, and many other countries.
5 Barlow and Durand (2009).
6 Bruce et al. (2005), table 2; for patients' experiences after recovery (for whatever reason) see their figure 2.
7 For references, see chapter 10.
8 Wolpert (1999). For his own experience, see especially the introduction and chapter 12. For other good descriptions of depression, see Solomon (2001) and Styron (2001). For a discussion of Abraham Lincoln's melancholia, see Shenk (2006).
9 Coleridge, "Dejection," quoted in Wolpert (1999), 8.
10 This is the mainstream view of psychiatrists. They do not view depression as an either/or phenomenon.

11 This is the system of classification known as DSM-V, DSM meaning Diagnostic and Statistical Manual.

12 At least four if you have not experienced both depressed mood and loss of interest.

13 For further analysis of the PHQ-9, see Kroenke, Spitzer, and Williams (2001). That paper, however, uses a more generous description: 5–9 Mild; 10–14 Moderate; 15–19 Moderately Severe; 20+ Severe. For evidence on frequency distributions in Germany, see Martin et al. (2006). On GAD, see Löwe et al. (2008) for a German population that shows 8% scoring 8 or more.

14 All the data we give on depression are based on Barlow and Durand (2009). As mentioned in chapter 3, it appears that depressions now start earlier in life than they used to.

15 Monroe and Harkness (2011).

16 Formerly known as manic-depression. On average such people experience some seventeen weeks of depression per year and some five weeks of mania (Judd et al. [2002]). During periods of mania or extreme depression, such people are considered to be in a psychotic state.

17 Barlow and Durand (2009), 217, col. 2. Because there are very many more people with unipolar depression, more suicide attempts come from people with unipolar than bipolar depression (see chapter 3).

18 Merikangas et al. (2011).

19 These do not include the cases of multiple personality, which is a rare form of personality disorder.

20 Williams (2001), 48.

21 Barlow and Durand (2009), 479.

22 DSM-V includes a number of other personality disorders as well, but the two types discussed here are in the words of McManus et al. (2009), "two types with particular public and mental health policy relevance."

23 UK Adult Psychiatric Morbidity Survey, 2007. Own calculations.

24 Coulthard et al. (2002), 23, 66, and 68.

25 For example, there is an unsettled argument about whether cannabis abuse can cause schizophrenia. However, even if it can, the effect must be small since schizophrenia has not increased in Britain over the last fifty years (Kirkbride et al. [2012]), while cannabis use has grown from zero to where nearly half of all twenty-five- to thirty-four-year-olds in Britain have tried it (McManus et al. [2009], 179). The Advisory Council on the Misuse of Drugs estimates that of 5,000 people taking cannabis, one might become schizophrenic as a result (ACMD [2008], 19). On alcoholism in the United States, see Barlow and Durand (2009), 398.

26 Kessler et al. (2005b), 620. On Britain, see McManus et al. (2009), where a similar number are severely or moderately dependent on alcohol.

27 In England every year 9,000 people die from alcohol-related deaths. Nearly 290,000 hospital admissions annually are wholly due to alcohol and 880,000 are partly attributable to alcohol. Both of these numbers more than doubled between 2002–3 and 2010–11 (Health and Social Care Information Centre [2012]).

28 Roy and Linnoila (1986). Note that this criterion is less demanding than the criterion used in ICD-10 (the International Classification of Disease, widely used in Europe) and DSM-IV used in the United States, which also require preoccupation and persistence despite evidence of harm.

29 Coulthard et al. (2002), 29, 69. Data for Britain. Also, half of them are alcohol dependent (own analysis of 2007 Psychiatric Morbidity Survey). In Britain altogether 2,000 people, nearly all men, die each year from taking hard drugs (mostly heroin and methadone) (BMA Board of Science [2013], 40–43).

30 McManus et al. (2009), chapter 11.

31 Kim-Cohen et al. (2003); Kessler et al. (2005a). Both sources, one from New Zealand and one from the United States, show that 50% of adults with mental illness experienced it before the age of fifteen. Since more adults experience mental illness than children, more than 50% of children who have mental illness will experience it as adults.

32 Green et al. (2005), 35.

33 Van Ameringen, Mancini, and Farvolden (2003).

34 Moffitt (1993; 2003).

35 On wider definitions, 5% of children worldwide have ADHD (Polanczyk et al. [2007]).

36 These areas are activated by the emotional aspects of physical pain as well as by mental pain generated by, for example, social exclusion (Eisenberger et al. [2003]), the sound of a crying baby (Lorberbaum et al. [1999]), or the physical pain of a loved one (Singer et al. [2004]). (Physical pain also has sensory components experienced in other parts of the brain that, according to Kross et al. [2011] are also affected by social exclusion.) Interestingly, it has also been shown that people who self-report greater pain from an unpleasant physical stimulus also report greater pain from the experience of social rejection in a laboratory experiment (Eisenberger et al. [2006]).

37 In the United States and Britain about 2% of all adults over sixteen have dementia.

Chapter 3. How Many Suffer?

1 The data on adults are as follows. United States: Kessler et al. (2005b) (1-year prevalence, 2011). Britain: McManus et al. (2009) (point prevalence, 2007). EU: Wittchen and Jacobi (2005) (1-year prevalence, meta-analysis for 2001–3), which draws on a range of studies including the WHO World Mental Health Surveys (2001–3), known in Europe as ESEMeD—see

Demyttenaere et al. (2004). For a range of individual country data, see annex 3. All data exclude dementia.

For children, see Global Burden of Disease Study 2010 (2012). (Reproduced in Layard and Hagell [2015], 9). Other estimates give higher numbers for the United States. The Centers for Disease Control and Prevention estimate a figure of 13–20% (Perou et al. [2013], annual prevalence).

2 See Kessler et al. (2005b) and annex 3, tables 3 and 4.

3 Based on the World Health Survey: see Ayuso-Mateos et al. (2010). Similar findings are in Rai et al. (2013). The World Mental Health Survey also showed the same levels of depression in developed and developing countries (Ferrari et al. [2013], 472). For individual country data, see annex 3. For special surveys in China, see Phillips et al. (2009)—they give a 1-month prevalence of any mental disorder of 18%.

On anxiety disorders, see a meta-analysis by Baxter et al. (2013), figure 2, who find a world rate of 7%. On schizophrenia, see Jablensky (2009).

4 See also Layard et al. (2013a), and Kessler and Üstün (2008).

5 Kessler et al. (2005a), table 2—which estimates 46% for the United States. The movement in and out of depression/anxiety can be judged from the follow-up of the British Psychiatric Morbidity Survey 2000 (Singleton and Lewis [2003]). In the eighteen-month follow-up, 8% were depressed/anxious throughout, 8% recovered (i.e., half), and 5% became new cases. Similarly, among children using a thirty-six-month follow-up, 4% who were initially well developed emotional disorders and 4% developed conduct disorders. At the same time 76% of children with emotional disorders recovered, as did 57% of children with conduct disorder (Meltzer et al. [2003])—based on a follow-up of the 1999 survey. All these results exaggerate the degree of movement (due to measurement error).

6　The number of households in England is 21 million. The number of adults with mental illness is about 7.5 million (McManus et al. [2009]). From the British Household Panel Survey we can infer that the number of households with at least one mentally ill adult is about 80% of the number of mentally ill people, i.e., about 6 million. In addition, many adults in households without any mentally ill adults will have a mentally ill child. And on top of this, many will have a mentally ill parent, living elsewhere.

7　Global Burden of Disease Study 2010 (2012). Perou et al. (2013) give a higher figure of 13–20% of children in the United States.

8　For example, Kessler et al. (1994).

9　For a general survey, see Fombonne (1995), 554–55. For example, in one Swedish district, Lundby, a careful study of the whole population showed significant increases in depression (severe or medium) between 1947 and 1957 and between 1957 and 1972 (Hagnell et al. [1990], 81–82, tables 48c and d). For longer-term changes in Britain, see Ferri, Bynner, and Wadsworth (2003).

10　For the United States, Kessler et al. (2005c). For Britain, Meltzer et al. (1995); Singleton et al. (2001); McManus et al. (2009).

11　Twenge et al. (2010). This is a meta-analysis of surveys using the Minnesota Multiphasic Personality Inventory. The authors examine the argument that later generations are less defensive in their responses but conclude that such response bias makes little difference to their results (151).

12　Layard and Dunn (2009), 3. See also Collishaw et al. (2004); Maughan et al. (2008).

13　West and Sweeting (2003).

14　Moussavi et al. (2007). In another study the World Mental Health Survey assesses the proportion of people who are severely disabled for (i) people with physical disorders (24% of them are severely disabled) and (ii) people with mental disorders (41% of them are severely disabled)—see Ormel et al. (2008), table 3.

15 See WHO (2008).

16 These figures relate to 2004, see WHO (2008). Since this assessment of the global burden of disease, which was endorsed by the WHO, there has been another assessment by the same authors published in the *Lancet* (380, December 2012). The new analysis gives the share of mental illness in overall morbidity in advanced countries as 28% (compared with 38%) and the share of musculoskeletal complaints at 25% (compared with 7%) (Vos et al. [2012]). The change is thought to reflect pressure from middle- and lower-income countries to treat musculoskeletal problems more seriously, since the same weights for each condition are applied in every country, regardless of the different significance of the condition at different levels of economic development. (Other changes since 2008 are that discounting has been abandoned, as has the use of a standard age distribution in every country.)

17 WHO (2008).

18 Twenty-nine percent of hospital inpatient and outpatient expenditure in England is in the last year of life (Seshamani and Gray [2004]).

19 Much of the analysis in this section is based on Williams (2001), chapters 2 and 3. In England in 2008, 4,530 deaths were recorded as suicide.

20 Barlow and Durand (2009), 251; Blumenthal (1988); Barraclough et al. (1974).

21 Williams (2001), 36.

22 WHO (2002), table 1.2.

23 People who attempt suicide or do violence to others are on average found to have lowered levels of serotonin. This is related to impulsivity (Williams [2001], 122). However, it is important to stress how difficult it is to predict suicide. For

evidence that greater availability of antidepressants reduces the level of suicide in a country, see Gusmão et al. (2013).

24 Williams (2001).

25 Storr (1990).

26 These are self-report figures. Hospital statistics give a figure more like 0.3%.

27 McManus et al. (2009). In addition a further 2.5% say they have self-harmed without intending to risk their lives. Much lower figures for attempted suicide are found in Belgium, France, Germany, Italy, the Netherlands, and Spain—an average of 1.3% (Bernal et al. [2007]).

28 About half of all successful suicides are by people who have already made a previous attempt (Isometsä and Lönnqvist [1998]).

29 Williams (2001).

Chapter 4. Do They Get Help?

1 Annex 3, table 5 and annex 4.

2 Ormel et al. (2008) based on the World Mental Health Surveys (see their table 1). For treatment rates for individual countries, see annex 3, table 5.

3 McManus et al. (2009), 47. Numbers in treatment in the past week. Data relate to 2007. At that point most of this treatment was not following NICE guidelines. Since then IAPT has expanded provision, and over the year 2012/13 provided two or more sessions to about 6% of people with depression and anxiety disorders (see chapter 12). But those in IAPT treatment at any point in time were only about 1.5% of people with depression and anxiety disorders.

In the European Union the comparable figures were 9% getting just medication and 11% getting psychological treatment (with or without medication)—see Wittchen and Jacobi (2005), table 5. A further 6% were seen but not treated.

4 On alcohol and drug problems there are also data directly from the UK National Drug Treatment Monitoring System. For people with alcohol as their primary problem, the National Treatment Agency in 2012/13 treated in total 110,000 people (of whom 76,000 were new cases). Nine thousand were treated in inpatient units and/or residential rehab. The median age was thirty-five. Nearly all clients (89%) were treated within three weeks. Seventy thousand left treatment, of whom 58% were no longer dependent on alcohol.

For people with drug problems, the National Treatment Agency in 2012–13 treated twice as many people as for alcohol problems—nearly 200,000 people (of whom 70,000 were new cases). Nine thousand were treated in inpatient units and/or residential rehab. A third of new cases had been on opiates only, and another quarter on opiates and crack cocaine. The median age was thirty-five. Nearly all clients were treated within three weeks. Sixty-two thousand left treatment, of whom a third were abstinent and another 13% free of dependency.

5 For the United States see Kataoka, Zhang, Wells (2002). British figures from Green et al. (2005).

6 Wang et al. (2005). See also Bruce et al. (2005).

7 National Confidential Inquiry into Suicide and Homicide by People with Mental Illness, NCISH (2013).

8 McHugh et al. (2013). See also Chilvers et al. (2001), Deacon and Abramowitz (2005), and van Schaik et al. (2004).

9 Cunningham (2009).

10 Ad hoc survey of RCGP members carried out in 2010. Five hundred and ninety members replied to the specific questions.

11 Thornicroft (2006). He recommends a three-pronged attack on knowledge, attitudes, and behavior.

12 www.time-to-change.org.uk. See also Henderson and Thornicroft (2013).

13 APPG on Mental Health (2008). Only ninety-four MPs replied.

14 Hansard, vol. 546, col. 504 et seq. (June 14, 2012).

Chapter 5. How Does It Affect People's Lives?

1 Layard (2011a), chapter 2.

2 See Helliwell, Layard, and Sachs (2012), chapter 3.

3 See annex 5.1. The analysis there includes multivariate analysis, with and without fixed person effects.

4 Dolan and Metcalfe (2012). See annex 5.2.

5 See annex 5.2.

6 Mykletun et al. (2009), tables 1 and 3. (The figures are, strictly, odds ratios.) Very few of these deaths were by suicide. The net effect of depression was unaffected when "smoking, alcohol and physical activity" were included as covariates. 4.9% were diagnosed as depressed.

7 In the United States, participants in the Framingham Heart Study took a depression scale test. Over the following six years the most depressed third were 88% more likely to die than the least depressed third, after allowing for age and sex (Wulsin et al. [2005]). In England, two studies have used the General Health Questionnaire (GHQ-12) as a measure of distress. Robinson, McBeth, and MacFarlane (2004) studied 4,500 adults in northwest England. Compared with the least disturbed third of people, the most disturbed third were 70% more likely to die each year over the following eight years (after allowing for age and sex). Similarly, Russ et al. (2012), table 3, used the Health Survey for England. Respondents in 1994–2004 were followed up for an average of eight years to ascertain their survival. At any age the 7% most mentally disturbed people had an annual probability of death that was 67% higher than the corresponding figure for the 60%

least disturbed, after fully allowing for their initial physical condition.

8 Data from Professor Andrew Steptoe of University College London. See also Steptoe and Wardle (2012) for earlier results.

9 Patten et al. (2008), table 1. On stroke, see also Pan et al. (2011), figure 3. On coronary heart disease, see also Nicholson, Kuper, and Hemingway (2006).

10 Chida et al. (2008). Such people were also more likely to die. (But the authors warn against possible bias, since positive findings are more likely to get published.) See also Satin, Linden, and Phillips (2009), who in their meta-analysis find depressed patients 39% more likely to die than other cancer patients.

11 Satin, Linden, and Phillips (2009).

12 See meta-analyses by Nicholson, Kuper, and Hemingway (2006) for depression, and by Roest et al. (2010) for anxiety. For hospital consultations by patients with asthma, see Ahmedani et al. (2013).

13 Thornicroft (2011).

14 See Jones, Howard, and Thornicroft (2008). For example, people with diabetes and comorbid mental illness who presented to an emergency department were less likely to be admitted to hospital for diabetic treatment.

15 Regier et al. (1990). In some studies these effects predominate, see Whooley et al. (2008).

16 McEwen (1998); Kiecolt-Glaser et al. (2002); Steptoe and Kivimäki (2012); Brotman, Golden, and Wittstein (2007). For the Whitehall II results, see Steptoe, Wardle, and Marmot (2005), and Steptoe et al. (2008).

17 Kumari et al. (2011).

18 Danese et al. (2007). The inflammation index is based on an aggregate of high-sensitivity C-reactive protein, fibrinogen, and white blood-cell count.

19 Boscarino (2004).

20 Kiecolt-Glaser et al. (1995) administered a small punch biopsy wound to more and less stressed subjects, and observed the rate of healing. Cole-King and Harding (2001) studied patients at a wound clinic and observed the effect of mood on the rate of healing (a "natural" experiment).

21 Cohen, Tyrrell, and Smith (1991) administered infectious nasal drops and observed the relationship between subsequent symptoms and initial stress.

22 Danese et al. (2007).

23 Nimnuan, Hotopf, and Wessely (2001). The clinics were dental, chest, rheumatology, cardiology, gastroenterology, neurology, and gynecology. In these clinics the patients with medically unexplained symptoms had average scores for anxiety (especially) and depression that were above the population average.

24 Bermingham et al. (2010).

25 We can distinguish the different directions of causality by carefully noting what precedes what.

26 Naylor et al. (2012), 4.

27 McManus et al. (2009). Special analysis.

28 On the United States, see Goetzel et al. (2004), table 2A, and Bureau of Labor Statistics, *Labor Force Statistics from the Current Population Survey 2014*, table 47. On other countries, see OECD (2012). Also note that according to Pauly et al. (2002) the costs of absenteeism far exceed the wages paid for days off sick.

29 On this point, according to the Sainsbury Centre for Mental Health (2007), 70 million days of absence are due to mental illness (8), of which 10.5 million are due to work-related mental illness (10) (Health Survey for England figures).

30 See, for example, Goetzel et al. (2004) and compare their tables 2A and 3A. See also Centre for Mental Health (2010). Presenteeism is partly reflected in lowered weekly earnings, but child mental illness also lowers educational performance, which is another source of lowered earnings.

31 Lundborg, Nilsson, and Rooth (2011).

32 Duckworth and Seligman (2005). The partial correlation co-efficients were 0.65 for resilience and 0.25 for IQ. See also Baumeister and Tierney (2011).

33 Drugs are a major cause of crime, with 14% of prisoners inside for a drug offense and 55% for offenses connected with their drug habit. Forty percent of prisoners were dependent on drugs in the year before going to prison. Alcohol is also a major problem, with 30% of sentenced men having severe alcohol dependency (Prison Reform Trust [2012], 57, 59).

34 James and Glaze (2006).

35 Singleton et al. (1998), 41, 95. Only 8% are psychotic (53).

36 Ten percent had been in a mental hospital at some point in their life (Singleton et al. [1998]).

37 A 59% reoffending rate for prisoners with mental health problems, compared with 50% for other prisoners (Cunniffe et al. [2012]).

38 Worell (2002).

39 Pettitt et al. (2013).

40 The analysis is for Britain and uses the British Cohort Study of people born in 1970; see Layard et al. (2013b). Life-satisfaction is measured by answers to the following question: "Here is a scale from 0 to 10. On it '0' means that you are completely dissatisfied and '10' means that you are completely satisfied. Please tick the box with the number above it which shows how dissatisfied or satisfied you are about the way your life has turned out so far."

41 Note that on its own, income explains under 1% of the variance of life-satisfaction across individuals, compared with 11% explained by all the factors taken together. The rest of the variation cannot be explained by factors we are able to measure.

42 A broad-minded economist is the Nobel Prize winner James Heckman. But until recently even his work on "noncogni-

tive skills" focused only on the skills that related to behavior: Heckman (2008).

43 Similar results are found from American data, using the Panel Study of Income Dynamics (PSID)—see Smith and Smith (2010). Using sibling fixed effects the authors find that psychological problems in childhood reduce education by 0.3 years, family income in adulthood by 29%, annual earnings by $5,300, weeks worked by seven weeks per year, and the probability of marriage by 11 percentage points.

Chapter 6. The Economic Cost

1 OECD (2012), 47. This defines mental illness as severe illness (the worst 5% in mental health) and moderate illness (the next 15%). The resulting reductions in total employment are 3.4% for the United States, 4.8% for Britain, and 3.7% on average for eight other OECD countries. Note that the concept of cost ideally compares the present with an alternative where mentally ill people had no mental illness but were otherwise the same as now.

2 OECD (2012), figure 4.2.

3 On the United States, see Goetzel et al. (2004), tables 1 and 2A. On Britain and continental Europe, see OECD (2012), 73.

4 Goetzel et al. (2004).

5 Centre for Mental Health (2010). It is also estimated that in 1999 alcohol and drug abuse cost the US economy about $200 billion (excluding the cost of death), i.e., 2% of GDP (US Department of Health and Human Services [2008]).

6 Sainsbury Centre for Mental Health (2009).

7 On the United States see Anderson (1999), and on United Kingdom, see Brand and Price (2000) and Sainsbury Centre for Mental Health (2009).

8 Scott et al. (2001). The figures are excess costs between ages ten and twenty-eight, discounted and expressed in 2012

prices. Note that this figure is roughly in line with "a half of 2% being borne by the taxpayer," since it is approximately 1% (£600,000 is the present value of output per person).

9   Friedli and Parsonage (2007).

10 Katon (2003); Hutter, Schnurr, and Baumeister (2010).

11 On the United States, see Levit et al. (2013), table 1. According to Frank (2011), table 1, the percentages in 2002–4 were USA 0.9%, UK 1.1%, Germany and France 1.0%, Canada and Australia 0.7%. For more recent data, see WHO Mental Health Atlas, and Garg and Evans (2011).

12 Levit et al. (2013), exhibit 1, 2009 figure.

13 We use an exchange rate of $1.5 to the £ (pound sterling) throughout this book.

14 Primary care support, psychological therapy in IAPT, and medication. For detail, see UK edition of this book.

15 Seshamani and Gray (2004).

16 At the world level, mental health research contributes only 3–4% of health literature (Saxena et al. [2006]).

17 Of total National Institute of Health disease-specific research in 2012, 7% went on schizophrenia, depression, and dementia. See Moses et al. (2015).

Chapter 7. What Causes Mental Illness?

1   Freud did however allow an important role for genetics, in producing the common elements in human nature and in producing a greater risk of illness in some people compared with others.

2   Heston (1966).

3   The rate of schizophrenia in the general population is around 1%. Heston's study used a small sample, but a large-scale Danish study confirms the results (Kety et al. [1994]).

4   There are traces of the idea in Aristotle (*De Anima*). For a powerful attack on the blank slate, see Pinker (2002).

5 This is still high since prevalence in the overall population is about 1%.

6 There is abundant evidence that the main reason is not a greater similarity of experience—see Plomin et al. (2013).

7 Plomin et al. (2013), passim.

8 This is based on correlational analysis, not identification of the specific genes. See Plomin et al. (2013), especially 252–54; Kendler et al. (1992); Kendler et al. (2003).

9 Plomin et al. (2013).

10 There is a major science that attempts to compute the "heritability" of different conditions, in other words to measure how much of the variation in a condition between people is due to differences in their genes. But this is not really possible where genes and environment interact (nor even if they are correlated)—see annex 7.

11 This is sometimes called the diathesis-stress model—diathesis being the inherited vulnerability, which interacts with the environmentally determined stressor.

12 Fagiolini et al. (1994).

13 Cadoret et al. (1995).

14 Bohman (1996); Sigvardsson, Bohman, and Cloninger (1996); Plomin et al. (2013),. 121.

15 Caspi et al. (2003). The graph shows the effect of bad life events in your twenties. Similar results are found about the effect of maltreatment as a child (their figure 2).

16 Hariri et al. (2002).

17 Bennett et al. (2002).

18 See Plomin et al. (2013), 124–25. See also Kendler et al. (1995). Moreover, bad genes can lead people into situations where bad events occur (McGuffin, Owen, and Gottesman [2004]).

19 IJzendoorn, Belsky, and Bakermans-Kranenburg (2012); refers only to Caucasian samples.

20 Eley et al. (2012).

21 Anisman et al. (1998).

22 Suomi (1997).

23 On the rest of this section, see Rutter (2000; 2004), and Rutter et al. (2008). We are also beginning to discover influences from life in the womb. For example, heavy drinking by the mother in the first three months risks "fetal alcohol syndrome," which can cause ADHD (Mattson, Crocker, and Nguyen [2011]).

24 Chapman et al. (2004). Our calculations.

25 Layard and Dunn (2009), 22–26.

26 Amato (2000).

27 Ford, Goodman, and Meltzer (2004), table 5, and Ford et al. (2007), table 3. Also Rutter (2000), 392.

28 Layard and Dunn (2009), 20–21.

29 Ford, Goodman, and Meltzer (2004); Ford et al. (2007); and Rutter et al. (1998).

30 Seligman (1992).

31 Brown and Harris (1978).

32 For an analysis of how pro-inflammatory cytokines produced in response to infection may induce depression, see Dantzer et al. (2008).

33 Naylor et al. (2012).

34 Lucas et al. (2004).

35 Lundberg and Cooper (2011).

36 Income is not asked about in the UK Adult Psychiatric Morbidity Survey.

37 Ford, Goodman, and Meltzer (2004), table 5, and Ford et al. (2007), table 3. Interestingly, children's life-satisfaction is also uncorrelated with income per head in the family (Knies [2012]).

38 Lund et al. (2011).

39 The odds of an event are its probability divided by (1 minus its probability). Thus for the high-risk group the odds are 1 and for the low-risk group the odds are 0.14.

40 Note that the numbers in this table are fairly typical of our ability to predict mental illness. In the table we can take risk to be a variable that is either 1 or 0, and mental illness to be a variable that is either 1 or 0. The correlation between these two variables is r = 0.375 with r^2 = 0.141.

41 Duffy et al. (2013). An even more powerful study used initial thinking style to predict psychological recovery from traffic accidents (Ehring, Ehlers, and Glucksman [2008]).

42 See Helliwell, Layard, and Sachs (2012), 50–52.

43 Ferrari et al. (2013), using World Mental Health Survey, and Ayuso-Mateos et al. (2010), using World Health Survey. See also Helliwell, Layard, and Sachs (2012), chapter 3, using Gallup World Poll data on negative affect. By contrast there is a relation between positive affect (or life-satisfaction) and national income per head. This is strongest when no other factors are included besides income (as in Stevenson and Wolfers [2008]). When other relevant factors are also included the effect falls greatly for life-satisfaction and disappears for positive affect (see Helliwell, Layard, and Sachs [2012], 64).

44 The partial correlation coefficients are, respectively, 0.35, 0.24, 0.23 (Helliwell, Layard, and Sachs [2012], 64). These were the only variables with significant effects. Income per head and healthy life expectancy had the expected signs but ill-determined effects. Analysis by John Helliwell.

45 Helliwell and Wang (2011).

46 James (2007), 343–44; James (2008). See also Wilkinson and Pickett (2009) for further pairwise correlations, which are discussed more fully in our chapter 15.

47 Helliwell (2003), 351, and Helliwell, Layard, and Sachs (2012), 71. See also Cruwys et al. (2014).

48 Marmot et al. (2010); Commission on Social Determinants of Health (2008).

Chapter 8. Does Therapy Work?

1 Mayou, Ehlers, and Hobbs (2000). For a survey of all available studies, see Rose et al. (2002).

2 See Morens (1999). Washington was relieved of five pints of blood in one day.

3 See T. D. Wilson (2011). Examples include Healthy Families America (to prevent child abuse), DARE (to reduce drug taking), Dollar a Day (to deter teenage pregnancy), Scared Straight and boot camps (to reduce delinquency), paying young people to improve school performance and school attendance, and most study skills programs. For more details, see chapter 15.

4 Wessely (2007).

5 Manson et al. (2003).

6 ECT has been shown to help with severe and persistent depression, and nonorganic catatonia.

7 Hollon, Thase, and Markowitz (2002).

8 Blanchflower and Oswald (2011) show that in Europe 8% have taken antidepressants in the last twelve months, including 4% who did so continuously for more than four weeks. On severity, see our annex 3, tables 3 and 5 (remembering that most treatment is pills).

9 Beck (1976).

10 See Evans (2012). This point was also stressed by Albert Ellis at roughly the same time as Beck began to stress it. It gave rise to his ABC model where the Activating event combines with our Beliefs to generate the Consequences. Ellis's history too is interesting. As a rather shy Jewish adolescent growing up in New York, he decided to treat his shyness with women by forcing himself to talk to a hundred women in the Bronx Botanical Gardens within a month. He eventually became a psychoanalyst. But after six years as an analyst, he began

to doubt its efficacy. People's mental health, he thought, depends not just on what happens to them but also on how they react. So to escape from depression and anxiety, you have to learn to master your thoughts, accept yourself and others, and love rather than be loved. By training people in this "rational therapy," Ellis claimed he could make them better. But he did not go on, as Beck did, to a scientific evaluation of his treatment. His many writings include *Reason and Emotion in Psychotherapy*.

11 Rush et al. (1977).
12 Dobson et al. (2008).
13 DeRubeis, Siegle, and Hollon (2008); Goldapple et al. (2004).
14 Durham et al. (2004); Ehlers et al. (2013); Franklin et al. (2000); Gillespie et al. (2002); Hahlweg et al. (2001); Lincoln et al. (2003); Merrill, Tolbert, and Wade (2003).
15 Franklin et al. (2000).
16 Ost (2009) summarized 189 studies that followed up patients with anxiety disorders who had been treated with CBT. The mean follow-up period was 2.1 years with some studies going up to 9 years. On average people were as well at follow-up as at the end of treatment, in each anxiety disorder.
17 Mörtberg, Clark, and Bejerot (2011).
18 Hollon et al. (2005); Dobson et al. (2008).
19 Teasdale et al. (2000).
20 Stiles et al. (2008). For a critique, see D. M. Clark, Fairburn, and Wessely (2008).
21 D. M. Clark (2011).
22 Royal College of Psychiatrists (2013).
23 D.M. Clark et al. (2006); Ehlers et al. (2014).
24 Grey et al. (2008).
25 Wampold et al. (1997).
26 The overall results are reported in Stangier et al. (2011).

Chapter 9. How Therapies Are Developed

1 Roth and Fonagy (2005).
2 Wolpe (1958).
3 Paul (1966).
4 Beck et al. (1979).
5 Rush et al. (1977).
6 Dobson et al. (2008).
7 Some practitioners prefer the term "cognitive therapy," since it emphasizes that all the techniques aim to help patients identify and change their negative beliefs.
8 Barlow and Durand (2009), 127.
9 Naipaul (1985), 3.
10 D. M. Clark (1986).
11 Ehlers and Breuer (1992).
12 Ehlers (1995).
13 NICE (2011c).
14 D. M. Clark et al. (1994).
15 NICE (2013d).
16 Katzelnick et al. (2001).
17 Van Ameringen, Mancini, and Farvolden (2003).
18 Katzelnick et al. (2001).
19 Wittchen et al. (1999).
20 Katzelnick et al. (2001).
21 Stein et al. (1999).
22 D. M. Clark and Wells (1995).
23 NICE (2013d).
24 D. M. Clark et al. (2006).
25 Stangier et al. (2011); Leichsenring et al. (2013); Mayo-Wilson et al. (2014).
26 Boecking (2010).

Chapter 10. What Works for Whom?

1 See chapter 2.

2 The relevant treatment guidelines for adult problems discussed in this chapter are: NICE (2004; 2005b; 2005c; 2009a; 2009b; 2009c; 2009d; 2011a; 2011c; 2013b; 2013d), except where otherwise stated. On children, see chapter 13.

3 Monroe and Harkness (2011).

4 Hollon et al. (2006).

5 Fava et al. (2004). In this experiment people who had recovered from depression with the help of imipramine medication were divided into two groups, one of which was given ten half-hour sessions of CBT. Neither group continued medication, unless they relapsed.

6 Segal, Williams, and Teasdale (2013).

7 D. M. Clark et al. (1994); D. M. Clark et al. (1998); D. M. Clark et al. (2006); Ehlers et al. (2010); Ehlers et al. (2014); Siev and Chambless (2007); NICE (2005b).

8 Siev and Chambless (2007).

9 D. M. Clark et al. (1994); Barlow et al. (2000).

10 D. M. Clark et al. (1997).

11 NICE (2013d).

12 Stangier et al. (2011); D. M. Clark et al. (2006); Leichsenring et al. (2013); Mayo-Wilson et al. (2014).

13 Mörtberg, Clark, and Bejerot (2011); Heimberg et al. (1993).

14 Leichsenring et al. (2013).

15 Ost, Fellenius, and Sterner (1991).

16 Gyani et al. (2013).

17 Ehring, Ehlers, and Glucksman (2008); Duffy et al. (2013).

18 Bisson et al. (1997); Mayou, Ehlers, and Hobbs (2000).

19 Fairburn, Marcus, and Wilson (1993).

20 G. T. Wilson and Fairburn (2007).

21 Agras et al. (2000).

22 Barlow et al. (2000).

23 G. T. Wilson and Fairburn (2007).

24 Ehlers et al. (2014).

25 D. M. Clark et al. (1999); D. M. Clark et al. (2014).

26 NICE (2004; 2005b; 2005c; 2009c; 2011c; 2013d).

27 D. M. Clark et al. (2009).

28 Gyani et al. (2013).

29 Kopelowicz, Liberman, and Zarate (2007).

30 Butzlaff and Hooley (1998).

31 Leff et al. (1982).

32 Giesen-Bloo et al. (2006).

33 Bateman and Fonagy (2009).

34 Linehan et al. (2006).

35 Nutt (2012).

36 NICE (2011a).

37 Csete (2010).

38 RIOTT (Randomized Injectable Opiate Treatment Trial). Britain also has a policy of free needle exchange, to control infection.

39 NICE (2007).

40 Fifty percent of people with criminal records in Britain are unemployed (Nutt [2012]).

41 See Domoslawski (2011).

42 This approach has increasing support. In 2011 it was proposed by the Global Commission on Drug Policy, which included among its members five former presidents or prime ministers and a former UN Secretary General (www.global commissionondrugs.org). The commission's report presents a good overview of the evidence (see also Babor et al. [2010]). In Britain the approach was endorsed by the All-Party Parliamentary Group on Drug Policy Reform (2013) chaired by Molly Meacher. The issue is now on the agenda of the Organization of American States. Meanwhile, in the United States, Colorado and Washington have legalized the sale of cannabis. Every policy has its pros and cons, but in this case the pros outweigh the cons by a very large margin.

43 Devilly and Borkovec (2000).

44 Kocsis et al. (2009). Patients were also offered the combination of both, and those who preferred the combination did best if that was what they got. On patient preference, see McHugh et al. (2013).

45 Ginzburg et al. (2012).

Chapter 11. Can We Afford More Therapy?

1 British data. Department of Health (DH) (2008b); NHS Confederation (2012), 3.

2 Katon (2003); Hutter, Schnurr, and Baumeister (2010); Naylor et al. (2012), 11.

3 Chiles et al. (1999), 209.

4 This is the cost of the system of stepped care used in England's Improving Access to Psychological Therapies Program (IAPT). The program involves a mixture of (i) high-intensity treatment, which costs nearer to $1,500, as mentioned in chapter 1, and (ii) low-intensity treatment, which is cheaper. The figure of $1,000 per person treated comes from taking IAPT expenditure in 2011–12 ($320 million) and dividing it by numbers treated (330,000). Unfortunately there are no later data on expenditure because the survey on investment in mental health was discontinued.

5 Work by Dr. Arek Hassy.

6 Howard et al. (2010). Cost data from Simon Dupont.

7 Moore et al. (2007). Cost data are in 1997 prices.

8 In another trial for people who have had heart attacks a clinical psychologist wrote a manual that included six weekly sections covering specific self-help treatments for intrusive and distressing thoughts, anxiety, depression, undue illness behavior, panic disorder, and other psychological problems heart-attack patients commonly experience (Lewin et al. [1992]). In the pilot study patients who had had heart attacks were

divided randomly into two groups when they left the hospital. Patients in the treatment group were given the manual, plus an exercise program and tapes on relaxation and stress management. The psychologist phoned them three times during the next six weeks in case they needed help. The control group was given standard handouts covering most of the same information and was also contacted three times in the same way. Yet over the next year those treated with the manualized program made on average three fewer visits to their primary care doctor and had 0.33 fewer hospitalizations. Since the program cost under £50 per patient, it clearly paid for itself.

9 Gulliksson et al. (2011).

10 There have been other studies in which CBT was less successful—most famously the so-called ENRICHD program (Berkman et al. [2003]). This gave a median of eleven sessions of individual CBT, beginning a median of seventeen days after the heart attack. One possible reason why this trial failed was that the treatment began too soon after the heart attack.

11 Ladapo et al. (2012).

12 Simon et al. (2007). See also Molosankwe et al. (2012) for a meta-analysis of results relating to diabetes, and Knapp, McDaid, and Parsonage (2011) for an application to Britain. On arthritis, see Sharpe et al. (2001), who, however, include no costs. There is now a whole new branch of medicine that deals with the mental health needs of physically ill people admitted to the hospital. It is called liaison psychiatry and can be extremely cost effective. For example, the City Hospital in Birmingham treats people with acute physical illness. In 2009 it introduced a service known as RAID (Rapid Assessment Interface and Discharge). This is directed at all emergency patients admitted for physical reasons but also showing signs of mental illness. There is a team of specialists who treat the patients, but they also train the whole staff of the hospital

about mental health issues. As a result patients stay less time in the hospital and come back in less frequently. The overall savings are estimated to be at least four times the extra cost of the service (Parsonage and Fossey [2011]).

13   Proudfoot et al. (1997).

14   In Britain both figures are approximately $1,000 (Department for Work and Pensions and note 4 above). See also Layard et al. (2007): the figure for Exchequer savings per month used there was $1,100, and the figure for the cost of treatment was $1,100. In the United States both figures are approximately $2,000.

15   Our calculation has to be about the numbers expected to be off benefit, but most of the evidence we have is about numbers back in work. Which of these numbers is bigger? Clearly some of those gaining work would not otherwise have been on benefits. But equally some people stop claiming benefit without going into work. It is likely that the second group exceeds the first since, when we compare mentally ill people with others, the difference in employment rates is less than the difference in the proportion on benefit (Layard et al. [2007], table 3). In the British context, evidence about effects on employment understates the effects on benefit dependence.

16   Fournier et al. (2014) (18% is the percentage of the original sample).

17   Wells et al. (2000).

18   Rollman et al. (2005).

19   Proudfoot et al. (1997). The sample was all unemployed people with nonmanual occupations. For an analysis using computerized CBT (cCBT) on a general sample of people with depression or anxiety, see McCrone et al. (2004): this found that the total cost of NHS resources (including the cost of the cCBT) was not significantly increased for the cCBT group, and there were major employment effects.

20 See annex 11.

21 In the IAPT program described in the next chapter, it is only possible to look at changes during the period of treatment, not over the following twenty-five months. The following table shows the proportion of those treated who during treatment left incapacity/sickness benefits, and the proportion who entered onto incapacity/sickness benefits.

	Left benefit	Entered benefit	Net change in number on benefit
Doncaster pilot	12%	8%	4%
Newham pilot	10%	4%	5%
IAPT 1st year	7%	5%	2%
IAPT 2012/13	7%		

It is the net change that matters, but it ought of course to be compared with a counterfactual, which would probably be an increase in numbers on benefit. And in principle a longer period of follow-up is desirable. Note that during treatment at least 45% of IAPT patients recover, as assumed in Layard et al. (2007). Sources: D. M. Clark et al. (2009) and IAPT records.

22 McManus et al. (2009).

Chapter 12. Improving Access to Psychological Therapies

1 McHugh et al. (2013). See also Chilvers et al. (2001); Deacon and Abramowitz (2005); and van Schaik et al. (2004).

2 The IAPT program's website is www.iapt.nhs.uk.

3 The paper was written by Richard Layard, based on intensive discussions with David Clark and Molly Meacher (Layard [2005]).

4 We have never found out who removed the word "cognitive" from an earlier draft of the manifesto.

5 LSE Centre for Economic Performance's Mental Health Policy Group (2006).

6 The implementation plan was published in February 2008 (Department of Health [2008a]). The next major document was published in February 2010 (Department of Health [2010]).

7 On the competences, see Roth and Pilling (2008). The training curricula were based on the manuals in the trials identified by NICE. The curricula also specified how clinical skills should be assessed, by rating therapist performance in videotapes of sessions and by written assignments (case reports and essays). Accreditation of training courses and trainees is provided through the British Association of Behavioural and Cognitive Therapists and the British Psychological Society.

8 This was for high-intensity therapists. Low-intensity therapists receive one day in college and four in practice.

9 Not more than two trainees per trained member of staff.

10 Census of the IAPT Workforce in 2014. Available from the IAPT website (www.iapt.nhs.uk)

11 This was helped by a campaign led by Mind. Mind and the other mental health charities have always given IAPT invaluable support.

12 Stiles et al. (2008).

13 Clark et al. (2009).

14 All IAPT services upload fifty data items per patient for central processing by the Health and Social Care Information Centre (HSCIC). IAPT Performance Reports of varying complexity are published by HSCIC at monthly, quarterly, and yearly intervals (see http://www.hscic.gov.uk/iaptmonthly). Data from these reports, and other sources, can be viewed on the World Wide Web by accessing the Public Health England's

Mental Health, Dementia & Neurology Intelligence Network's Common Mental Health Disorders Profiles (Fingertips) Tool, http://fingertips.phe.org.uk/profile-group/mental-health/profile/common-mental-disorders. The website includes a downloadable user guide that explains how to change between the various data views in the Fingertips Tool. The data can also be downloaded for offline analysis.

15 Health and Social Care Information Centre (2014).

16 See the report on the first three years (Department of Health [2012]).

17 The concept of recovery here is very specific. Before each session of treatment every patient completes two brief questionnaires. One is the PHQ-9, which assesses depression and is shown in chapter 2. The other is a well-validated measure of anxiety. In many cases the anxiety measure is the GAD-7 shown in chapter 2. However, for some anxiety disorders (such as social anxiety, PTSD, obsessive-compulsive disorder) questionnaires more closely tailored to that specific condition are preferred. Details of these questionnaires can be found in the IAPT Minimum Data Set (MDS), which can be downloaded from the IAPT website, www.iapt.nhs.uk. A patient is considered to be "diagnosable" if before treatment she scored above the cut-off for either depression or anxiety or both (nearly all the patients who are treated are diagnosable). They are then considered to have recovered if at the last session of treatment they are below the cut-off on *both* questionnaires. This concept of recovery is stricter than in most published clinical trials, which generally only require people to have recovered on one measure (depression or anxiety). It has the advantage that it is simple to understand, but it only provides a partial picture of the benefits of IAPT. For some people recovery may require a very small change, while other people who are really ill when they come into

treatment may improve a lot without "recovering." So IAPT also reports whether the patient has "reliably improved"—that is, they have improved more than could occur through chance. On that criterion, around two-thirds of IAPT patients reliably improve (Gyani et al. [2013]). And only 8% reliably deteriorate—fewer than would be found in any comparable untreated group.

18 D. M. Clark (2009).

19 However, the response rates in the follow-up were not high (36% in Newham and 51% in Doncaster).

20 Variation in IAPT performance by local area (termed clinical commissioning group or CCG) for a wide range of indexes (access, recovery, reliable improvement, wait times, pre- and posttreatment data completeness, completeness of ICD-10 codes, etc.) can be viewed on the World Wide Web by accessing the Public Health England's Mental Health, Dementia & Neurology Intelligence Network's Common Mental Health Disorders Profiles (Fingertips) Tool, http://fingertips.phe.org.uk /profile-group/mental-health/profile/common-mental-disorders. Each index can be viewed in multiple ways (by area from highest to lowest performing; across time within an area; comparing areas with their neighbors geographically or in terms of social deprivation, ethnicity, etc.).

21 HSCIC's Quarterly IAPT performance report for July to September 2014 showed that IAPT services in fifty-nine health areas (termed "clinical commissioning groups, CCGs") exceeded 50% recovery, nineteen health areas exceeded 55% recovery, and five health areas exceeded 60%. There are 211 health areas (CCGs) in England.

22 Gyani et al. (2013). The findings that follow do not of course reflect random assignment.

23 In addition, return to work is more frequent where step-up rates are higher.

24 Pimm and Virathajenman (2015).

25 With at least 60% of therapists giving high-intensity treatment.

26 In fact the services are exceeding this target. Data published by the Health and Social Care Information Centre in 2014 showed that on average IAPT services had pre- to posttreatment data completeness for 96.8% of people who had received a course of treatment (i.e., two or more sessions). As far as we are aware, this level of complete outcome data has never been achieved in large mental health systems anywhere in the world. Such high levels of data completeness are also rare in randomized controlled trials.

27 Year 1 data.

28 D. M. Clark et al. (2009).

29 Now called clinical commissioning groups.

30 Census of the IAPT Workforce in 2014. Available from the IAPT website, www.iapt.nhs.uk.

31 Griffiths and Steen (2013b). In a separate paper, Griffiths and Steen (2013a) claim that IAPT is costing more than anticipated. This is wrong. The simplest way to work out cost is to divide total expenditure by numbers treated. For 2011–12 this gives £650 per course of treatment compared to the original estimate of £750. The authors disregard these numbers and try to calculate the cost of a session of therapy, rather than a course. Unfortunately, this is impossible as no information is available on the number of sessions in 2011–12. It is also not relevant since the main issue is the relation between overall cost and outcomes (regardless of the number of sessions).

32 This is similar to the early experience of the National Health Service; see Timmins (2001).

33 Health and Social Care Information Centre (2014).

34 HM Government/Department of Health (2011).

35 Older people have never been excluded from the program, but they are currently underrepresented.

36 The Adult Psychiatric Morbidity Survey (McManus et al. [2007]) showed that only 42% of mentally ill people on incapacity benefits were in treatment for their condition (private tabulation).

37 It is also very important to have earlier interventions before people reach incapacity benefits—i.e., while people still have jobs but are off sick. The British government is introducing a "Health and work assessment and advisory service" for employers and employees, when employees have been off sick for more than four weeks (Department for Work and Pensions [2013]). There are many useful strategies that therapists can follow at this stage. For example, workers who have been off sick may need graded exposure and a gradual return to work, beginning as soon as possible. In one experiment the patients of CBT therapists trained in employment issues returned to full-time work sixty-five days earlier than patients receiving regular CBT (Lagerveld et al. [2012]).

38 President's New Freedom Commission on Mental Health (2003).

39 On US mental health policy, see Frank and Glied (2006).

40 Karlin and Cross (2014).

41 Karlin et al. (2010).

42 Karlin et al. (2012).

43 Karlin et al. (2013).

44 See correspondence in October 2014 issue of *American Psychologist*.

Chapter 13. What Works for Young People?

1 Quoted in Layard and Dunn (2009), 113.

2 Kennedy (2010).

3 See Layard and Hagell (2015). See also chapter 3 above.

4 Green et al. (2005), tables 5.11 and 6.11. See also Ford et al. (2007).

5   Kessler et al. (2005a) and Kim-Cohen et al. (2003).

6   This is true of most but not all conditions. It is true of conduct disorder, but for social phobia success rates are higher among adults than children. With very early intervention there is also the risk that the treatment is wasted if given too soon, before there is evidence that the problem will not cure itself. The rates of spontaneous recovery from mental illness are higher among children than among adults (see chapter 3, note 5), and there is no clear evidence that successful treatment of children produces effects that last longer than successful treatment of adults. On the other hand children's ability to learn and thus succeed in later life depends crucially on being mentally healthy as a child (Van Ameringen, Mancini, and Farvolden [2003]).

7   Friedli and Parsonage (2007). Present value at age eight.

8   For example, Cohen and Piquero (2009) take those 4% of men who have the highest number of police contacts between the ages of fourteen and twenty-six. They estimate the average present value of their cost to society as between $2.6 million and double that.

9   For a survey, see Wolpert et al. (2006).

10 NICE has clinical guidelines expressly for children on depression (NICE [2005a]), ADHD (NICE [2013c]), autism (NICE [2011b]), and antisocial behavior and conduct disorders (NICE [2013a]), and guidelines that include children with PTSD (NICE [2005c]), obsessive-compulsive disorder (NICE [2005b]), panic disorder and generalized anxiety disorder (NICE [2011c]), and social anxiety disorder (NICE [2013d]).

11 Barrett, Dadds, and Rapee (1996). This compares with 30% in the wait-list group. Recovery was maintained after twelve months.

12 Chapter by Fonagy and Target in Roth and Fonagy (2005).

13 Webster-Stratton and Reid (2010). Their main program is designed for children age two to eight. The Triple P Program

also offers parent training for parents of teenagers (Sanders, Markie-Dadds, and Turner [2003]).

14 Scott, Briskman, and O'Connor (2014). But using teachers' reports and the reports of the children themselves, there was no longer an effect on school behavior—the fading issue discussed in the next chapter. The study is known as SPACE (Study of Parents' and Adolescents' Experiences). Good results were also found from an integrated program of targeting behavior and reading. This SPOKES program is evaluated in Scott et al. (2010).

15 Lochman, Wells, and Lenhart (2008). For a highly readable manual for parents, see Kazdin (2009).

16 Roth and Fonagy (2005), 396.

17 Chapter by Fonagy and Target in Roth and Fonagy (2005).

18 NICE (2013c).

19 Weiss et al. (2005); Meade and Steiner (2010). See chapter 8, note 3.

20 See Kelvin, Layard, and York (2009), 15.

21 Layard and Hagell (2015).

Chapter 14. Can We Prevent Mental Illness?

1 See Olds et al. (1998); Lee et al. (2012); and Eckenrode et al. (2010).

2 For surveys of the evidence, see Weare and Nind (2011); McDaid and Park (2011); Substance Abuse and Mental Health Services Administration (2007); and World Health Organization (2004). For cost-effectiveness studies, see Lee et al. (2012), and Knapp, McDaid, and Parsonage (2011).

3 Many quite famous programs have had at least one comprehensive trial giving no positive outcome. These include beyondblue (Sawyer et al. [2010]); Triple P (Little et al. [2012], Eisner et al. [2012]); Resourceful Adolescent Program (Stallard et al. [2012]); the Incredible Years on subclinical groups

of children as opposed to those with diagnoses (Scott, Briskman, and O'Connor [2014]).

4 Parks (2000) and Heckman et al. (2010).

5 T. D. Wilson (2011), 215.

6 Kellam et al. (2008), and Ialongo et al. (1999). The program covered some five hundred hours of school time.

7 For example, suppose there is an intervention that actually makes no difference. If it is used in hundreds of experiments on randomly selected participants drawn from some large population, the intervention will be judged statistically significant in 5% of the experiments (assuming the criterion of significance used is the 5% level). The same would also be true if we studied hundreds of different interventions, all of which had no effect.

8 For most of the main clinical treatments discussed earlier in the book, there have been such meta-analyses.

9 Durlak et al. (2011). All used a control group, but only half were randomized. The results were similar for the randomized and nonrandomized controls (personal correspondence with Durlak).

10 For similar findings, see also two analyses of PATHS (Promoting Alternative Thinking Strategies): Conduct Problems Prevention Research Group (2011), table 3; and Conduct Problems Prevention Research Group (2010); and also the analysis of the UK Penn Resiliency Program by Challen, Machin, and Gillam (2013).

11 Goleman (1996; 2006).

12 Humphrey, Lendrum, and Wigelsworth (2010). There is, however, good evidence within the group of schools doing SEAL that good implementation produced better results (Banerjee, Weare, and Farr [2014]). As regards primary SEAL there has been no controlled experiment involving children's outcomes—but see Hallam, Rhamie, and Shaw (2006), and Gross (2010).

13 On this and the next paragraph, see T. D. Wilson (2011).

14 See, for example, Challen, Machin, and Gillam (2013) and many other studies that include follow-up data.

15 *Nicomachean Ethics.*

16 The PATHS program is one exception that lasts a lot longer. It includes 130 lessons over a one-year period. See, for example, Kelly et al. (2004); Curtis and Norgate (2007).

17 Weare and Nind (2011).

18 The program was devised after a worldwide search reported in Hale, Coleman, and Layard (2011). The programs drawn on include the Penn Resiliency Program, Media Navigator, Mindfulness in Schools (b), Academic Possible Selves, Unplugged, Relationship Smarts, SHAHRP, Science of Mental Health, Mood Gym, Parents under Construction.

19 Bailey (2013).

20 Seligman (2011).

21 Brunwasser, Gillham, and Kim (2009); Challen, Machin, and Gillam (2013).

22 For encouraging preliminary results, see Harms et al. (2013).

23 The best informal introductions to mindfulness are by the Vietnamese master Thich Nhat Hanh (Hanh [2008; 2001]). For a scholarly introduction, see Williams and Kabat-Zinn (2013); and for a practical self-help guide, see Williams and Penman (2011). See also Huffington (2014).

24 We are talking here of nonclinical groups. The use of mindfulness-based cognitive therapy (MBCT) for patients recently recovered from depression was discussed in chapter 10.

25 Baer (2003). Shorter courses also have effects (Weng et al. [2013]).

26 Hölzel et al. (2011). It also increases telomerase, conducive to longer life (Jacobs et al. [2011]).

27 Davidson et al. (2003).

28 On US marines, see Stanley and Jha (2009). On children and young people, see Harnett and Dawe (2012); Burke (2010);

Raes et al. (2013); Huppert and Johnson (2010); Weare (2012); and Schonert-Reichl and Lawlor (2010).

29 Weare (2012).

30 In a recent survey of teachers in British schools and colleges, 54% said behavior was worse than five years ago and only 7% said it was better (Association of Teachers and Lecturers [2013]). Some 35% of staff said they did not get training in how to deal with challenging, disruptive, or violent students.

31 Benson (2006).

32 S. Wilson et al. (2007). In a British national survey, "Understanding Society," children ages ten to fifteen were asked how often other children misbehaved in class. Some 27% said "in most classes" and 47% said "in over half of all classes" (Knies [2012], appendix 1). This significantly reduced their life-satisfaction (appendix 2).

33 British data. Neill (2008).

34 Webster-Stratton et al. (2011); Reinke et al. (2012); Davenport and Tansey (2009); Webster-Stratton et al. (2001).

35 Baker-Henningham et al. (2012); Hutchings et al. (2007).

36 For Head Start, see T. D. Wilson (2011). In Britain, the Sure Start Program, begun in 1999, had much less structured ways of working than most interventions. There was also no randomized evaluation. However, comparing Sure Start with similarly deprived non–Sure Start areas suggested that Sure Start significantly improved five out of fourteen outcomes at the age of three (Melhuish et al. [2008]). By the age of seven rather fewer significant effects were observed, but for three out of eight outcomes where changes were measured between three and seven there were significant effects (Department for Education [2012]).

37 Knapp McDaid, and Parsonage (2011), 4–5.

38 Durlak et al. (2011), 420. In some states, like Illinois, it is all schools.

39 Ofsted (2013), 20. Ofsted estimated that 40% of the teaching of life skills needed improving.

40 Layard and Hagell (2015).

Chapter 15. Would a Better Culture Help?

1 Layard, Mayraz, and Nickell (2010); Helliwell, Layard, and Sachs (2012), chapter 3.

2 Layard (2011a), 81.

3 For fuller treatments of the topics in this chapter, see Layard (2011a; 2009; 2011b).

4 For a justification of this approach, see Layard (2011a), chapter 15. For the view that this approach is too one-dimensional, see Sen (2009) and Skidelsky and Skidelsky (2012).

5 See, for example, the program called Parents under Construction.

6 See Cowan and Cowan (2000).

7 National Family and Parenting Institute (2000).

8 Layard (2011a), 16.

9 World Economic Forum (2012). See also Sennett (2003).

10 Deci and Ryan (1985), and Lundberg and Cooper (2011).

11 Layard (2011a), 156–60.

12 Robertson and Cooper (2011).

13 Edmans (2011).

14 http://positivenews.org.uk/2012/culture/media/9085/news-doesnt-reflect-real-world-newsreader-martyn-lewis/.

15 Leveson (2012). Prior to Leveson the main codes of conduct for printed material in Britain were (i) the one administered by the Press Complaints Commission applying to the responsibilities of editors and publishers, and (ii) the one administered by the National Union of Journalists (NUJ), which defined the conditions where the NUJ would defend a member against their employer.

16 This would obviously not cover classified ads.

17 Marmot et al. (2004).

18 Letter to the Republican Citizens of Washington County, Maryland (1809).

19 Layard (2011a), chapter 15. See also O'Donnell et al. (2014).

20 On Bhutan and Britain, see Helliwell, Layard, and Sachs (2012), chapters 5 and 6. On OECD, see OECD (2013), and O'Donnell et al. (2014).

21 See chapter 5 and annex 5.1.

22 Knies (2012). This study also examines the effect of specific items of child deprivation. They do have some effect, but much less than family relationships and social activity. And they cannot be mainly determined by income, since if they were, income itself would have an effect.

23 See chapter 7.

24 Lucas (2003).

25 The strongest argument for this is Kahneman's findings about loss aversion (Kahneman [2011]), together with the findings about the ineffectiveness of economic growth in increasing happiness (e.g., Helliwell, Layard, and Sachs [2012], chapter 3). See also De Keulenaer et al. (2014).

26 Layard et al. (2008). See also Stevenson and Wolfers (2010).

27 Wilkinson and Pickett (2009), 183. They also show two time series. But none of the relationships show how inequality affects outcomes, when other possible influences are also taken into account.

28 Helliwell, Layard, and Sachs (2012), 71.

29 B. Wilson (2008).

30 Seligman (2002; 2011).

31 In the United States a national government survey of complementary and alternative medicine found that 9% of respondents had used meditation in the past twelve months: http://nccam.nih.gov/sites/nccam.nih.gov/files/news/nhsr12.pdf.

32 The website is actionforhappiness.org.

33 For the effect of religion on happiness, see Helliwell, Layard, and Sachs (2012), 71–72.

Chapter 16. Stop This Pain

1 In the United Kingdom the annual average cost of treating a diabetic patient is €2,697 (Kanavos, van den Aardweg, and Schurer [2012], appendix 5).

2 L. Donnelly, "Lord Tebbit's Wife Margaret: Norman and I Don't Have Time to Cry," *The Telegraph*, November 22, 2009.

3 In the United States, the Mental Health Parity Act (MHPA), 1996, and the Mental Health Parity and Addiction Equality Act, 2008, require parity of treatment in insurance policies for mental and physical health (if both are covered) but do not require that a policy cover both. In England, see the Health and Social Care Act 2012, clause 1.

4 Rutz, von Knorring, and Walinder (1992). After a while the rates rose again as the trained doctors left the island.

5 A look at the NHS Outcomes Framework 2014–15, which is the cornerstone of the Mandate for NHS England, does not suggest that it was determined in that way.

6 British Association for Counselling and Psychotherapy (2010).

7 For evidence on declining violence and its cultural roots, see Pinker (2011). For data on crime in England and Wales, see Crime Survey for England and Wales—Office for National Statistics, Home Office.

REFERENCES

Advisory Council on the Misuse of Drugs (ACMD). 2008. *Cannabis: Classification and Public Health*. London: Home Office.

Agras, W. S., B. T. Walsh, C. G. Fairburn, G. T. Wilson, and H. C. Kraemer. 2000. "A Multicenter Comparison of Cognitive Behavioral Therapy and Interpersonal Psychotherapy for Bulimia Nervosa." *Archives of General Psychiatry* 57 (5): 459–66.

Ahmedani, B. K., E. L. Peterson, K. E. Wells, and L. K. Williams. 2013. "Examining the Relationship between Depression and Asthma Exacerbations in a Prospective Follow-Up Study." *Psychosomatic Medicine* 75 (3): 305–10.

All-Party Parliamentary Group on Drug Policy Reform. 2013. "Towards a Safer Drug Policy: Challenges and Opportunities Arising from 'Legal Highs.'" London: All-Party Parliamentary Group on Drug Policy Reform. Available at http://www.drug policyreform.net/p/inquiry.html.

All-Party Parliamentary Group on Mental Health. 2008. *Mental Health in Parliament*. London: All-Party Parliamentary Group on Mental Health, Supported by the Royal College of Psychiatrists, Mind, Rethink and Stand to Reason.

Amato, P. R. 2000. "The Consequences of Divorce for Adults and Children." *Journal of Marriage and Family* 62 (4): 1269–87.

Anderson, D. A. 1999. "The Aggregate Burden of Crime." Available at Social Science Research Network (SSRN), http//ssrn.com /abstract=147911.

Anisman, H., M. D. Zaharia, M. J. Meaney, and Z. Merali. 1998. "Do Early-Life Events Permanently Alter Behavioral and Hormonal Responses to Stressors?" *International Journal of Developmental Neuroscience* 16 (3–4): 149–64.

Association of Teachers and Lecturers (ATL). 2013. *Press Release— Disruptive Behaviour in Schools and Colleges Rises alongside Increase in Children with Behavioural and Mental Health Problems.* Association of Teachers and Lecturers' Survey.

Ayuso-Mateos, J. L., R. Nuevo, E. Verdes, N. Naidoo, and S. Chatterji. 2010. "From Depressive Symptoms to Depressive Disorders: The Relevance of Thresholds." *British Journal of Psychiatry* 196: 365–71.

Babor, T. F., J. Caulkins, J., G. Edwards, B. Fischer, D. Foxcroft, K. Humphreys, . . . J. Strang. 2010. *Drug Policy and the Public Good.* Oxford: Oxford University Press.

Baer, R. A. 2003. "Mindfulness Training as a Clinical Intervention: A Conceptual and Empirical Review." *Clinical Psychology: Science and Practice* 10 (2): 125–43.

Bailey, L. 2013. *Developing Healthy Minds in Teenagers Project— Briefing Paper.* How to Thrive.

Baker-Henningham, H., S. Scott, K. Jones, and S. Walker. 2012. "Reducing Child Conduct Problems and Promoting Social Skills in a Middle-Income Country: Cluster Randomised Controlled Trial." *British Journal of Psychiatry* 201: 101–8.

Banerjee, R., K. Weare, and W. Farr. 2014. "Working with 'Social and Emotional Aspects of Learning' (SEAL): Associations with School Ethos, Pupil Social Experiences, Attendance, and Attainment." *British Educational Research Journal* 40: 718–42.

Barlow, D. H., and V. M. Durand. 2009. *Abnormal Psychology: An Integrative Approach.* 5th ed. Belmont, CA: Wadsworth Cengage Learning.

Barlow, D. H., J. M. Gorman, M. K. Shear, and S. W. Woods. 2000. "Cognitive Behavioral Therapy, Imipramine, or Their Combination for Panic Disorder: A Randomized Controlled Trial." *JAMA* 283: 2529–36.

Barraclough, B., J. Bunch, B. Nelson, and P. Sainsbury. 1974. "A Hundred Cases of Suicide: Clinical Aspects." *British Journal of Psychiatry* 125: 355–73.

Barrett, P. M., M. R. Dadds, and R. M. Rapee. 1996. "Family Treatment of Childhood Anxiety: A Controlled Trial." *Journal of Consulting and Clinical Psychology* 64 (2): 333–42.

Bateman, A., and P. Fonagy. 2009. "Randomized Controlled Trial of Outpatient Mentalization-Based Treatment versus Structured Clinical Management for Borderline Personality Disorder." *American Journal of Psychiatry* 166: 1355–64.

Baumeister, R. F., and J. Tierney. 2011. *Willpower: Rediscovering Our Greatest Strength*. New York: Penguin.

Baxter, A. J., K. M. Scott, T. Vos, and H. A. Whiteford. 2013. "Global Prevalence of Anxiety Disorders: A Systematic Review and Meta-Regression." *Psychological Medicine* 43 (5): 897–910.

Beck, A. T. 1976 *Cognitive Therapy and the Emotional Disorders*. New York: International Universities Press.

———. 2006. "How an Anomalous Finding Led to a New System of Psychotherapy." *Nature Medicine* 12 (10): 1139–41.

Beck, A. T., A. J. Rush, B. F. Shaw, and G. Emery. 1979. *Cognitive Therapy of Depression*. New York: Guilford Press.

Bennett, A. J., K. P. Lesch, A. Heils, J. C. Long, J. G. Lorenz, S. E. Shoaf, . . . J. D. Higley. 2002. "Early Experience and Serotonin Transporter Gene Variation Interact to Influence Primate CNS Function." *Molecular Psychiatry* 7 (1): 118–22.

Benson, P. L. 2006. *All Kids Are Our Kids: What Communities Must Do to Raise Caring and Responsible Children and Adolescents*. 2nd ed. San Francisco: Jossey-Bass.

Berkman, L. F., J. Blumenthal, M. Burg, R. M. Carney, D. Catellier, J. M. Cowan, . . . Enhancing Recovery in Coronary Heart Disease Patients Investigators (ENRICHD). 2003. "Effects of Treating Depression and Low Perceived Social Support on Clinical Events after Myocardial Infarction: The Enhancing Recovery in Coronary Heart Disease Patients (ENRICHD) Randomized Trial." *JAMA* 289 (23): 3106–16.

Bermingham, S., A. Cohen, J. Hague, and M. Parsonage. 2010. "The Cost of Somatisation among the Working-Age Population in England for the Year 2008–2009." *Mental Health in Family Medicine* 7: 71–84.

Bernal, M., J. M. Haro, S. Bernert, T. Brugha, R. de Graaf, R. Bruffaerts, . . . the ESEMED/MHEDEA Investigators. 2007. "Risk Factors for Suicidality in Europe: Results from the ESEMED Study." *Journal of Affective Disorders* 101: 27–34.

Bisson, J. I., P. L. Jenkins, J. Alexander, and C. Bannister. 1997. "Randomised Controlled Trial of Psychological Debriefing for Victims of Acute Burn Trauma." *British Journal of Psychiatry* 171: 78–81.

Blanchflower, D. G., and A. J. Oswald. 2011. "Antidepressants and Age." IZA Discussion Paper No. 5785.

Blumenthal, S. J. 1988. "Suicide: A Guide to Risk Factors, Assessment, and Treatment of Suicidal Patients." *Medical Clinics of North America* 72: 937–71.

BMA Board of Science. 2013. *Drugs of Dependence: The Role of Medical Professionals*. London: British Medical Association (BMA).

Boecking, B. 2010. "Mechanisms of Change in Cognitive Therapy for Social Phobia." PhD thesis, Institute of Psychiatry, King's College London, University of London.

Bohman, M. 1996. "Predisposition to Criminality: Swedish Adoption Studies in Retrospect." In *Genetics of Criminal and Antisocial Behaviour*, edited by G. Bock and J. Goode. Chichester, UK: John Wiley. CIBA Foundation Symposium 194.

Boscarino, J. A. 2004. "Posttraumatic Stress Disorder and Physical Illness: Results from Clinical and Epidemiologic Studies." *Annals of the New York Academy of Sciences* 1032: 141–53.

Brand, S., and R. Price. 2000. *The Economic and Social Costs of Crime*. Home Office Research Study 217. London: Home Office.

British Association for Counselling and Psychotherapy (BACP). 2010. *Attitudes to Counselling and Psychotherapy Report*. London: British Association for Counselling and Psychotherapy.

Brotman, D. J., S. H. Golden, and I. S. Wittstein. 2007. "The Cardiovascular Toll of Stress." *Lancet* 370 (9592): 1089–100.

Brown, G. W., and T. O. Harris. 1978. *Social Origins of Depression: A Study of Psychiatric Disorder in Women*. London: Tavistock.

Bruce, S. E., K. A. Yonkers, M. W. Otto, J. L. Eisen, R. B. Weisberg, M. Pagano, . . . M. B. Keller. 2005. "Influence of Psychiatric Comorbidity on Recovery and Recurrence in Generalized Anxiety Disorder, Social Phobia, and Panic Disorder: A 12-Year Prospective Study." *American Journal of Psychiatry* 162 (6): 1179–87.

Brunwasser, S. M., J. E. Gillham, and E. S. Kim. 2009. "A Meta-Analytic Review of the Penn Resiliency Program's Effect on Depressive Symptoms." *Journal of Consulting and Clinical Psychology* 77 (6): 1042–54.

Burke, C. A. 2010. "Mindfulness-Based Approaches with Children and Adolescents: A Preliminary Review of Current Research in an Emergent Field." *Journal of Child and Family Studies* 19 (2): 133–44.

Butzlaff, R. L., and J. M. Hooley. 1998. "Expressed Emotion and Psychiatric Relapse: A Meta-Analysis." *Archives of Psychiatry* 55: 547–52.

Cadoret, R. J., W. R. Yates, E. Troughton, G. Woodworth, and M. A. Stewart. 1995. "Genetic-Environmental Interaction in the Genesis of Aggressivity and Conduct Disorders." *Archives of General Psychiatry* 52 (11): 916–24.

Caspi, A., K. Sugden, T. E. Moffitt, A. Taylor, I. W. Craig, H. Harrington, . . . R. Poulton. 2003. "Influence of Life Stress on Depression: Moderation by a Polymorphism in the 5-HTT Gene." *Science* 301 (5631): 386–89.

Centre for Mental Health. 2010. *The Economic and Social Costs of Mental Health Problems in 2009/10*. London: Centre for Mental Health.

Challen, A. R., S. J. Machin, and J. E. Gillam. 2013. "The UK Resilience Programme: A School-Based Universal Non-Randomized Pragmatic Controlled Trial." *Journal of Consulting and Clinical Psychology* (advance online publication November 18, 2013).

Chapman, D. P., C. L. Whitfield, V. J. Felitti, S. R. Dube, V. J. Edwards, and R. F. Anda. 2004. "Adverse Childhood Experiences and the Risk of Depressive Disorders in Adulthood." *Journal of Affective Disorders* 82 (2): 217–25.

Chida, Y., M. Hamer, J. Wardle, and A. Steptoe. 2008. "Do Stress-Related Psychosocial Factors Contribute to Cancer Incidence and Survival?" *Nature Clinical Practice (Oncology)* 5 (8): 466–75.

Chiles, J. A., M. J. Lambert, and A. L. Hatch. 1999. "The Impact of Psychological Interventions on Medical Cost Offset: A Meta-Analytic Review." *Clinical Psychology: Science and Practice* 6 (2): 204–20.

Chilvers, C., M. Dewey, K. Fielding, V. Gretton, P. Miller, B. Palmer, . . . Glynn Harrison for the Counselling versus Antidepressants in Primary Care Study Group. 2001. "Antidepressant Drugs and Generic Counselling for Treatment of Major Depression in Primary Care: Randomised Trial with Patient Preference Arms." *British Medical Journal* 322: 1–5.

Clark, A. E., S. Flèche, and C. Senik. 2013. "The Great Happiness Moderation." In *Happiness and Economic Growth: Lessons from Developing Countries*, edited by A. E. Clark and C. Senik. Oxford: Oxford University Press.

Clark, D. M. 1986. "A Cognitive Approach to Panic." *Behaviour Research and Therapy* 24 (4): 461–70.

———. 2011. "Implementing NICE Guidelines for the Psychological Treatment of Depression and Anxiety Disorders: The IAPT Experience." *International Review of Psychiatry* 23: 318–27.

Clark, D. M., A. Ehlers, A. Hackmann, F. McManus, M.J.V. Fennell, N. Grey, . . . J. Wild. 2006. "Cognitive Therapy versus Exposure and Applied Relaxation in Social Phobia: A Randomised Controlled Trial." *Journal of Consulting and Clinical Psychology* 74 (3): 568–78.

Clark, D. M., C. G. Fairburn, and S. Wessely. 2008. "Psychological Treatment Outcomes in Routine NHS Services: A Commentary on Stiles et al. (2007)." *Psychological Medicine* 38 (5): 629–34.

Clark, D. M., R. Layard, R. Smithies, D. A. Richards, R. Suckling, and B. Wright. 2009. "Improving Access to Psychological Therapy: Initial Evaluation of Two UK Demonstration Sites." *Behaviour Research and Therapy* 47 (11): 910–20.

Clark, D. M., P. M. Salkovskis, E. Breitholtz, B. E. Westling, L. G. Ost, K. A. Koehler, . . . M. G. Gelder. 1997. "Misinterpretation of Body Sensations in Panic Disorder." *Journal of Consulting and Clinical Psychology* 65 (2): 203–13.

Clark, D. M., P. M. Salkovskis, A. Hackmann, H. Middleton, P. Anastasiades, and M. Gelder. 1994. "A Comparison of Cognitive Therapy, Applied Relaxation and Imipramine in the Treatment of Panic Disorder." *British Journal of Psychiatry* 164 (6): 759–69.

Clark, D. M., P. M. Salkovskis, A. Hackmann, A. Wells, M. Fennell, J. Ludgate, . . . M. G. Gelder. 1998. "Two Psychological Treatments for Hypochondriasis: A Randomised Controlled Trial." *British Journal of Psychiatry* 173 (3): 218–25.

Clark, D. M., P. M. Salkovskis, A. Hackmann, A. Wells, J. Ludgate, and M. Gelder. 1999. "Brief Cognitive Therapy for Panic Disorder: A Randomized Controlled Trial." *Journal of Consulting and Clinical Psychology* 67 (4): 583–89.

Clark, D. M., and A. Wells. 1995. "A Cognitive Model of Social Phobia." In *Social Phobia: Diagnosis, Assessment, and Treatment*, edited by R. Heimberg, M. Liebowitz, D. A. Hope, and F. R. Schneier, 69–93. New York: Guilford Press.

Clark, D. M., J. Wild, J. Grey, R. Stott, S. Liness, A. Deale, . . . A. Ehlers. 2014. "Doubling the Clinical Benefit of Each Hour of Psychotherapy: A Randomized Controlled Trial of Self-Study Assisted Cognitive Therapy for Social Anxiety Disorder." Manuscript submitted for publication.

Cohen, M. A., and A. R. Piquero. 2009. "New Evidence on the Monetary Value of Saving a High Risk Youth." *Journal of Quantitative Criminology* 25: 25–49.

Cohen, S., D.A.J. Tyrrell, and A. P. Smith. 1991. "Psychological

Stress and Susceptibility to the Common Cold." *New England Journal of Medicine* 325 (9): 606–12.

Cole-King, A., and K. G. Harding. 2001. "Psychological Factors and Delayed Healing in Chronic Wounds." *Psychosomatic Medicine* 63: 216–20.

Collishaw, S., B. Maughan, R. Goodman, and A. Pickles. 2004. "Time Trends in Adolescent Mental Health." *Journal of Child Psychology and Psychiatry* 45 (8): 1350–62.

Commission on Social Determinants of Health (CSDH). 2008. *Closing the Gap in a Generation: Health Equity through Action on the Social Determinants of Health*. Final Report of the Commission on Social Determinants of Health. Geneva: World Health Organization.

Conduct Problems Prevention Research Group (CPPRG). 2010. "The Effects of a Multiyear Universal Social-Emotional Learning Program: The Role of Student and School Characteristics." *Journal of Consulting and Clinical Psychology* 78 (2): 156–68.

———. 2011. "The Effects of the Fast Track Preventive Intervention on the Development of Conduct Disorder across Childhood." *Child Development* 82 (1): 331–45.

Cooper, K., and K. Stewart. 2013. *Does Money Affect Children's Outcomes? A Systematic Review*. York: Joseph Rowntree Foundation.

Coulthard, M., M. Farrell, N. Singleton, and H. Meltzer. 2002. *Tobacco, Alcohol, and Drug Use and Mental Health*. Office for National Statistics (ONS). London: The Stationery Office (TSO).

Cowan, C. P., and P. A. Cowan. 2000. *When Partners Become Parents: The Big Life Change for Couples*. Mahwah, NJ: Lawrence Erlbaum.

Cruwys, T., S. A. Haslam, G. A. Dingle, C. Haslam, and J. Jetten. 2014. "Depression and Social Identity: An Integrative Review." *Personality and Social Psychology Review* 18 (3): 215–38.

Csete, J. 2010. *From the Mountaintops: What the World Can Learn from Drug Policy Change in Switzerland*. Global Drug Policy Program. New York: Open Society Foundations.

Cunniffe, C., R. Van de Kerckhove, K. Williams, and K. Hopkins. 2012. *Estimating the Prevalence of Disability amongst Prisoners: Results from the Surveying Prisoner Crime Reduction (SPCR) Survey*. London: Ministry of Justice.

Cunningham, P. J. 2009. "Beyond Parity: Primary Care Physicians' Perspectives on Access to Mental Health Care." *Health Affairs* 28 (3): w490–w501.

Curtis, C., and R. Norgate. 2007. "An Evaluation of the Promoting Alternative Thinking Strategies Curriculum at Key Stage 1." *Educational Psychology in Practice* 23 (1): 33–44.

Danese, A., C. M. Pariante, A. Caspi, A. Taylor, and R. Poulton. 2007. "Childhood Maltreatment Predicts Adult Inflammation in a Life-Course Study." *Proceedings of the National Academy of Sciences (PNAS)* 104 (4): 1319–24.

Dantzer, R., J. C. O'Connor, G. G. Freund, R. W. Johnson, and K. W. Kelley. 2008. "From Inflammation to Sickness and Depression: When the Immune System Subjugates the Brain." *Nature Reviews Neuroscience* 9 (1): 46–56.

Davenport, J., and A. Tansey. 2009. "Outcomes of an Incredible Years Classroom Management Programme with Teachers from Multiple Schools." Trinity College Dublin / National Educational Psychological Service.

Davidson, R. J., J. Kabat-Zinn, J. Schumacher, M. Rosenkranz, D. Muller, S. F. Santorelli, . . . J. F. Sheridan. 2003. "Alterations in Brain and Immune Function Produced by Mindfulness Meditation." *Psychosomatic Medicine* 65: 564–70.

Deacon, B. J., and J. S. Abramowitz. 2005. "Patients' Perceptions of Pharmacological and Cognitive Behavioral Treatments for Anxiety Disorders." *Behavior Therapy* 36: 139–45.

Deci, E. L., and R. M. Ryan. 1985. *Intrinsic Motivation and Self-Determination in Human Behavior*. New York: Plenum.

De Keulenaer, F., J,-E. De Neve, G. Kavetsos, M. I. Norton, B. Van Landeghem, and G. W. Ward. 2014. "Individual Experience of

Positive and Negative Growth Is Asymmetric: Evidence from Subjective Well-Being Data." CEP Discussion Paper No. 1304. London: LSE Centre for Economic Performance.

Demyttenaere, K., R. Bruffaerts, J. Posada-Villa, I. Gasquet, V. Kovess, J. P. Lepine, . . . WHO World Mental Health Survey Consortium. 2004. "Prevalence, Severity, and Unmet Need for Treatment of Mental Disorders in the World Health Organization World Mental Health Surveys." *JAMA* 291 (21): 2581–90.

Department for Education (DfE). 2012. *The Impact of Sure Start Local Programmes on Seven Year Olds and Their Families*. National Evaluation of Sure Start Team, Research Report DFE-RR220. London: Department for Education.

Department for Work and Pensions (DWP). 2013. *Fitness for Work: The Government Response to "Health at Work—An Independent Review of Sickness Absence."* London: The Stationery Office (TSO).

Department of Health (DH). 2008a. *Improving Access to Psychological Therapies—Implementation Plan: National Guidelines for Regional Delivery*. London: Department of Health.

———. 2008b. *Raising the Profile of Long-Term Conditions Care: A Compendium of Information* (Gateway Reference 8734). London: Department of Health/Long Term Conditions team.

———. 2010. *Realising the Benefits: IAPT at Full Roll Out*. London: Department of Health.

———. 2011. *No Health without Mental Health: A Cross-Government Mental Health Outcomes Strategy for People of All Ages*. London: Department of Health.

———. 2012. *IAPT Three-Year Report: The First Million Patients*. London: Department of Health.

DeRubeis, R. J., G. J. Siegle, and S. D. Hollon. 2008. "Cognitive Therapy versus Medication for Depression: Treatment Outcomes and Neural Mechanisms." *Nature Reviews Neuroscience* 9: 788–96.

Devilly, G. J., and T. D. Borkovec. 2000. "Psychometric Properties of the Credibility/Expectancy Questionnaire." *Journal of Behavior Therapy and Experimental Psychiatry* 31: 73–86.

Dobson, K. S., S. D. Hollon, S. Dimidjian, K. B. Schmaling, R. J. Kohlenberg, R. Gallop, . . . N. S. Jacobson. 2008. "Randomized Trial of Behavioral Activation, Cognitive Therapy, and Antidepressant Medication in the Prevention of Relapse and Recurrence in Major Depression." *Journal of Consulting and Clinical Psychology* 76 (3): 468–77.

Dolan, P., and R. Metcalfe. 2012. "Valuing Health: A Brief Report on Subjective Well-Being versus Preferences." *Medical Decision Making* 32 (4): 578–82.

Domoslawski, A. 2011. *Drug Policy in Portugal: The Benefits of Decriminalizing Drug Use.* Global Drug Policy Program. New York: Open Society Foundations.

Duckworth, A. L., and M. E. Seligman. 2005. "Self-Discipline Outdoes IQ in Predicting Academic Performance of Adolescents." *Psychological Science* 16 (12): 939–44.

Duffy, M., D. Bolton, K. Gillespie, A. Ehlers, and D. M. Clark. 2013. "A Community Study of the Psychological Effects of the Omagh Car Bomb on Adults." *PLoS ONE* 8 (9): e76618.

Durham, R. C., P. L. Fisher, M.G.T. Dow, D. Sharp, K. G. Power, J. S. Swan, and R. V. Morton. 2004. "Cognitive Behaviour Therapy for Good and Poor Prognosis Generalized Anxiety Disorder: A Clinical Effectiveness Study." *Clinical Psychology and Psychotherapy* 11 (3): 145–57.

Durlak, J. A., R. P. Weissberg, A. B. Dymnicki, R. D. Taylor, and K. B. Schellinger. 2011. "The Impact of Enhancing Students' Social and Emotional Learning: A Meta-Analysis of School-Based Universal Interventions." *Child Development* 82 (1): 405–32.

Eckenrode, J., M. Campa, D. W. Luckey, C. R. Henderson, R. Cole, H. Kitzman, . . . D. Olds. 2010. "Long-Term Effects of Prenatal and Infancy Nurse Home Visitation on the Life Course of Youths: 19-Year Follow-Up of a Randomized Trial." *Archives of Pediatrics and Adolescent Medicine* 164 (1): 9–15.

Edmans, A. 2011. "Does the Stock Market Fully Value Intangibles?

Employee Satisfaction and Equity Prices." *Journal of Financial Economics* 101: 621–40.

Ehlers, A. 1995. "A 1-Year Prospective Study of Panic Attacks: Clinical Course and Factors Associated with Maintenance." *Journal of Abnormal Psychology* 104 (1): 164–72.

Ehlers, A., J. Bisson, D. M. Clark, M. Creamer, S. Pilling, D. Richards, . . . W. Yule. 2010. "Do All Psychological Treatments Really Work the Same in Posttraumatic Stress Disorder?" *Clinical Psychology Review* 30 (2): 269–76.

Ehlers, A., and P. Breuer. 1992. "Increased Cardiac Awareness in Panic Disorder." *Journal of Abnormal Psychology* 101 (3): 371–82.

Ehlers, A., A. Hackmann, N. Grey, J. Wild, S. Liness, I. Albert, A. Deale, R. Stott, and D. M. Clark. 2014. "A Randomized Controlled Trial of Intensive and Weekly Cognitive Therapy versus Emotion Focussed Supportive Therapy." *American Journal of Psychiatry*, 171, 294–304.

Ehlers, A., N. Grey, J. Wild, R. Stott, S. Liness, A. Deale, . . . D. M. Clark. 2013. "Implementation of Cognitive Therapy for PTSD in Routine Clinical Care: Effectiveness and Moderators of Outcome in a Consecutive Sample." *Behaviour Research and Therapy* 51 (11): 742–52.

Ehring, T., A. Ehlers, and E. Glucksman. 2008. "Do Cognitive Models Help in Predicting the Severity of Posttraumatic Stress Disorder, Phobia, and Depression after Motor Vehicle Accidents? A Prospective Longitudinal Study." *Journal of Consulting and Clinical Psychology* 76 (2): 219–30.

Eisenberger, N. I., J. M. Jarcho, M. D. Lieberman, and B. D. Naliboff. 2006. "An Experimental Study of Shared Sensitivity to Physical Pain and Social Rejection." *Pain* 126: 132–38.

Eisenberger, N. I., M. D. Lieberman, and K. D. Williams. 2003. "Does Rejection Hurt? An fMRI Study of Social Exclusion." *Science* 302: 290–92.

Eisner, M., D. Nagin, D. Ribeaud, and T. Malti. 2012. "Effects of a Universal Parenting Program for Highly Adherent Parents:

A Propensity Score Matching Approach." *Prevention Science* 13 (3): 252–66.

Eley, T. C., J. L. Hudson, C. Creswell, M. Tropeano, K. J. Lester, P. Cooper, . . . D. A. Collier. 2012. "Therapygenetics: The 5HTTLPR and Response to Psychological Therapy." *Molecular Psychiatry* 17 (3): 236–37.

European Commission. 2008. *Mental Health in the EU: Key Facts, Figures, and Activities*. Luxembourg: European Commission Directorate-General for Health and Consumers.

Evans, J. 2012. *Philosophy for Life: And Other Dangerous Situations*. London: Ebury Publishing.

Fagiolini, M., T. Pizzorusso, N. Berardi, L. Domenici, and L. Maffei. 1994. "Functional Postnatal Development of the Rat Primary Visual Cortex and the Role of Visual Experience: Dark Rearing and Monocular Deprivation." *Vision Research* 34 (6): 709–20.

Fairburn, G. G., M. D. Marcus, and G. T. Wilson. 1993. "Cognitive Behaviour Therapy for Binge Eating and Bulimia Nervosa: A Comprehensive Treatment Manual." In *Binge Eating: Nature, Assessment, and Treatment*, edited by C. G. Fairburn and G. T. Wilson, 361–404. New York: Guilford Press.

Fava, G. A., C. Ruini, C. Rafanelli, L. Finos, S. Conti, and S. Grandi. 2004. "Six-Year Outcome of Cognitive Behavior Therapy for Prevention of Recurrent Depression." *American Journal of Psychiatry* 161 (10): 1872–76.

Fergusson, D. M., L. J. Horwood, and E. M. Ridder. 2005. "Show Me the Child at Seven: The Consequences of Conduct Problems in Childhood for Psychosocial Functioning in Adulthood." *Journal of Child Psychology and Psychiatry* 46 (8): 837–49.

Ferrari, A. J., A. J. Somerville, A. J. Baxter, R. Norman, S. B. Patten, T. Vos, and H. A. Whiteford. 2013. "Global Variation in the Prevalence and Incidence of Major Depressive Disorder: A Systematic Review of the Epidemiological Literature." *Psychological Medicine* 43: 471–81.

Ferri, E., J. M. Bynner, and M.E.J. Wadsworth, eds. 2003. *Changing Britain, Changing Lives: Three Generations at the Turn of the Century*. London: Institute of Education, University of London.

Flèche, S., and R. Layard. 2015. "Do More of Those in Misery Suffer from Poverty, Unemployment or Mental Illness?" CEP Discussion Paper No. 1356. London: LSE Centre for Economic Performance.

Fombonne, E. 1995. "Depressive Disorders: Time Trends and Possible Explanatory Mechanisms." In *Psychosocial Disorders in Young People: Time Trends and Their Causes*, edited by M. Rutter and D. J. Smith, 616–85. Chichester, UK: John Wiley.

Ford, T., S. Collishaw, H. Meltzer, and R. Goodman. 2007. "A Prospective Study of Childhood Psychopathology: Independent Predictors of Change over Three Years." *Social Psychiatry and Psychiatric Epidemiology* 42 (12): 953–61.

Ford, T., R. Goodman, and H. Meltzer. 2004 "The Relative Importance of Child, Family, School, and Neighbourhood Correlates of Childhood Psychiatric Disorder." *Social Psychiatry and Psychiatric Epidemiology* 39 (6): 487–96.

Fournier, J. C., R. J. DeRubeis, J. Amsterdam, R. C. Shelton, and S. D. Hollon. 2014. "Gains in Employment Status Following Antidepressant Medication or Cognitive Therapy for Depression." *British Journal of Psychiatry*.

Frank, R. G. 2011. "Economics and Mental Health: An International Perspective." In *The Oxford Handbook of Health Economics*, edited by S. Glied and P. C. Smith. New York: Oxford University Press.

Frank, R. G., and S. Glied. 2006. *Better But Not Well*. Baltimore, MD: Johns Hopkins University Press.

Franklin, M. E., J. S. Abramowitz, J. T. Levitt, M. J. Kozak, and E. B. Foa. 2000. "Effectiveness of Exposure and Ritual Prevention for Obsessive-Compulsive Disorder: Randomized Compared with Nonrandomized Samples." *Journal of Consulting and Clinical Psychology* 68 (4): 594–602.

Frederick, S., and G. Loewenstein. 1999. "Hedonic Adaptation." In *Well-Being: The Foundations of Hedonic Psychology*, edited by D. Kahneman, E. Diener, and N. Schwarz, 302–29. New York: The Russell Sage Foundation.

Friedli, L., and M. Parsonage. 2007. *Mental Health Promotion: Building an Economic Case*. Belfast: Northern Ireland Association for Mental Health (NIAMH).

Garg, C. C., and D. B. Evans. 2011. *What Is the Impact of Non-Communicable Diseases on National Health Expenditures: A Synthesis of Available Data*. Discussion Paper No. 3. Geneva: World Health Organization.

Giesen-Bloo, J., R. van Dyck, P. Spinhoven, W. van Tilburg, C. Dirksen, T. van Asselt, . . . A. Arntz. 2006. "Outpatient Psychotherapy for Borderline Personality Disorder: Randomized Trial of Schema-Focused Therapy vs Transference-Focused Psychotherapy." *Archives of General Psychiatry* 63 (6): 649–58.

Gillespie, K., M. Duffy, A. Hackmann, and D. M. Clark. 2002. "Community Based Cognitive Therapy in the Treatment of Post-Traumatic Stress Disorder Following the Omagh Bomb." *Behaviour Research and Therapy* 40 (4): 345–57.

Ginzburg, D. M., C. Bohn, V. Hofling, F. Weck, D. M. Clark, and U. Stangier. 2012. "Treatment Specific Competence Predicts Outcome in Cognitive Therapy for Social Anxiety Disorder." *Behaviour Research and Therapy* 50 (12): 747–52.

Global Burden of Disease Study 2010. 2012. *Global Burden of Diseases, Injuries, and Risk Factors Study 2010*. Seattle: Institute for Health, Metrics, and Evaluation.

Goetzel, R. Z., S. R. Long, R. J. Ozminkowski, K. Hawkins, S. Wang, and W. Lynch. 2004. "Health, Absence, Disability, and Presenteeism Cost Estimates of Certain Physical and Mental Health Conditions Affecting US Employers." *Journal of Occupational and Environmental Medicine* 46 (4): 398–412.

Goldapple, K., Z. V. Segal, C. Garson, M. Lau, P. Bieling, S. Kennedy, and H. Mayberg. 2004. "Modulation of Cortical-Limbic Pathways: Treatment-Specific Effects of Cognitive Behavior Therapy." *Archives of General Psychiatry* 61: 34–41.

Goleman, D. 1996. *Emotional Intelligence: Why It Can Matter More than IQ.* London: Bloomsbury.

———. 2006. *Social Intelligence: The New Science of Human Relationships.* London: Hutchinson.

Green, H., A. McGinnity, H. Meltzer, T. Ford, and R. Goodman. 2005. *Mental Health of Children and Young People in Great Britain, 2004.* Office for National Statistics. Basingstoke: Palgrave Macmillan.

Grey, N., P. Salkovskis, A. Quigley, D. M. Clark, and A. Ehlers. 2008. "Dissemination of Cognitive Therapy for Panic Disorder in Primary Care." *Behavioural and Cognitive Psychotherapy* 36: 509–20.

Griffiths, S., and S. Steen. 2013a. "Improving Access to Psychological Therapies (IAPT) Programme: Scrutinising IAPT Cost Estimates to Support Effective Commissioning." *Journal of Psychological Therapies in Primary Care* 2 (2): 142–56.

———. 2013b. "Improving Access to Psychological Therapies (IAPT) Programme: Setting Key Performance Indicators in a More Robust Context: A New Perspective." *Journal of Psychological Therapies in Primary Care* 2 (2): 133–41.

Gross, J. 2010. "SEAL: The Big Experiment." *Better: Evidence-Based Education* 2 (2): 6–7.

Gulliksson, M., G. Burell, B. Vessby, L. Lundin, H. Toss, and K. Svärdsudd. 2011. "Randomized Controlled Trial of Cognitive Behavioral Therapy vs Standard Treatment to Prevent Recurrent Cardiovascular Events in Patients with Coronary Heart Disease." *Archives of Internal Medicine* 171 (2): 134–40.

Gusmão, R., S. Quintão, D. McDaid, E. Arensman, C. Van Audenhove, C. Coffey, ... U. Hegerl. 2013. "Antidepressant Utilization and Suicide in Europe: An Ecological Multi-National Study." *PLoS ONE* 8 (6): e66455.

Gyani, A., R. Shafran, R. Layard, and D. M. Clark. 2013. "Enhancing Recovery Rates: Lessons from Year One of IAPT." *Behaviour Research and Therapy* 51 (9): 597–606.

Hagnell, O., E. Essen-Möller, J. Lanke, L. Öjesjö, and B. Rorsman. 1990. *The Incidence of Mental Illness over a Quarter of a Century: The Lundby Longitudinal Study of Mental Illness in a Total Population Based on 42,000 Observation Years.* Stockholm: Almqvist and Wiksell International.

Hahlweg, K., W. Fiegenbaum, M. Frank, B. Schroeder, and I. von Witzleben. 2001. "Short- and Long-Term Effectiveness of an Empirically Supported Treatment for Agoraphobia." *Journal of Consulting and Clinical Psychology* 69 (3): 375–82.

Hale, D., J. Coleman, and R. Layard. 2011. "A Model for the Delivery of Evidence-Based PSHE (Personal Wellbeing) in Secondary Schools." CEP Discussion Paper No. 1071. London: LSE Centre for Economic Performance.

Hallam, S., J. Rhamie, and J. Shaw. 2006. *Evaluation of the Primary Behaviour and Attendance Pilot.* Research Report RR717. London: Department for Education and Skills.

Hanh, T. N. 2001. *Anger: Buddhist Wisdom for Cooling the Flames.* London: Rider.

———. 2008 *The Miracle of Mindfulness: The Classic Guide to Meditation,* reprint. London: Rider.

Hansard, vol. 546, col. 504 et seq. (June 14, 2012).

Hariri, A. R., V. S. Mattay, A. Tessitore, B. Kolachana, F. Fera, D. Goldman, . . . D. R. Weinberger. 2002. "Serotonin Transporter Genetic Variation and the Response of the Human Amygdala." *Science* 297 (5580): 400–403.

Harms, P. D., M. N. Herian, D. V. Krasikova, A. Vanhove, and P. B. Lester. 2013. *The Comprehensive Soldier and Family Fitness Program Evaluation—Report #4: Evaluation of Resilience Training and Mental and Behavioral Health Outcomes.* Comprehensive Soldier and Family Fitness and the Research Facilitation Team.

Harnett, P. H., and S. Dawe. 2012. "Review: The Contribution of

Mindfulness-Based Therapies for Children and Families and Proposed Conceptual Integration." *Child and Adolescent Mental Health* 17 (4): 195–208.

Health and Social Care Information Centre (HSCIC). 2012. *Statistics on Alcohol: England, 2012*. Health and Social Care Information Centre, Lifestyles Statistics.

———. 2014. *Psychological Therapies, Annual Report on the Use of IAPT Services: England 2013/14 Experimental Statistics*. Health and Social Care Information Centre.

Heckman, J. J. 2008. "Schools, Skills, and Synapses." *Economic Inquiry* 46 (3): 289–324.

Heckman, J. J., S. H. Moon, R. Pinto, P. A. Savelyev, and A. Yavitz. 2010. "The Rate of Return to the HighScope Perry Preschool Program." *Journal of Public Economics* 94 (1–2): 114–28.

Heimberg, R. G., D. G. Salzman, C. S. Holt, and K. A. Blendell. 1993. "Cognitive Behavioural Group Treatment for Social Phobia: Effectiveness at 5-Year Follow-Up." *Cognitive Therapy and Research* 17: 325–39.

Helliwell, J. F. 2003. "How's Life? Combining Individual and National Variables to Explain Subjective Well-Being." *Economic Modelling* 20 (2): 331–60.

Helliwell, J. F., and S. Wang. 2011. "Trust and Wellbeing." *International Journal of Wellbeing* 1 (1): 42–78.

Helliwell, J. F., R. Layard, and J. Sachs, eds. 2012. *World Happiness Report*. New York: The Earth Institute, Columbia University.

———. 2013. *World Happiness Report 2013*. New York: UN Sustainable Development Solutions Network.

Henderson, C., and G. Thornicroft. 2013. "Reducing Stigma and Discrimination: Evaluation of England's Time to Change Programme." *British Journal of Psychiatry* 202 (S55).

Heston, L. L. 1966. "Psychiatric Disorders in Foster Home Reared Children of Schizophrenic Mothers." *British Journal of Psychiatry* 112: 819–25.

Hollon, S. D., R. J. De Rubeis, R. C. Shelton, J. D. Amsterdam,

R. M. Salomon, J. P. O'Reardon, M. L. Lovett, P. R. Young, K. L. Haman, B. B. Freeman, and R. Gallop. 2005. "Prevention of Relapse Following Cognitive Therapy vs Medications in Moderate to Severe Depression." *Archives of General Psychiatry* 62 (4): 417–22.

Hollon, S. D., M. O. Stewart, and D. Strunk. 2006. "Enduring Effects for Cognitive Behavior Therapy in the Treatment of Depression and Anxiety." *Annual Review of Psychology* 57: 285–315.

Hollon, S. D., M. E. Thase, and J. C. Markowitz. 2002. "Treatment and Prevention of Depression." *Psychological Science in the Public Interest* 3 (2): 39–77.

Hölzel, B. K., J. Carmody, M. Vangel, C. Congleton, S. M. Yerramsetti, T. Gard, and S. W. Lazar. 2011. "Mindfulness Practice Leads to Increases in Regional Brain Gray Matter Density." *Psychiatry Research: Neuroimaging* 191 (1): 36–43.

Howard, C., S. Dupont, B. Haselden, J. Lynch, and P. Wills. 2010. "The Effectiveness of a Group Cognitive Behavioural Breathlessness Intervention on Health Status, Mood, and Hospital Admissions in Elderly Patients with Chronic Obstructive Pulmonary Disease." *Psychology, Health & Medicine* 15 (4): 371–85.

Huffington, A. 2014. *Thrive: The Third Metric to Redefining Success and Creating a Happier Life*. London: W. H. Allen.

Humphrey, N., A. Lendrum, and M. Wigelsworth. 2010. *Social and Emotional Aspects of Learning (SEAL) Programme in Secondary Schools: National Evaluation*. Research Report DFE-RR049. London: Department for Education.

Huppert, F. A., and D. M. Johnson. 2010. "A Controlled Trial of Mindfulness Training in Schools: The Importance of Practice for an Impact on Well-Being." *Journal of Positive Psychology* 5 (4): 264–74.

Hutchings, J., D. Daley, K. Jones, P. Martin, T. Bywater, and R. Gwyn. 2007. "Early Results from Developing and Researching the Webster-Stratton Incredible Years Teacher Classroom Management Training Programme in North West Wales." *Journal of Children's Services* 2 (3): 15–26.

Hutter, N., A. Schnurr, and H. Baumeister. 2010. "Healthcare Costs in Patients with Diabetes Mellitus and Comorbid Mental Disorders—A Systematic Review." *Diabetologia* 53: 2470–79.

Ialongo, N. S., L. Werthamer, S. G. Kellam, C. H. Brown, S. Wang, and Y. Lin. 1999. "Proximal Impact of Two First-Grade Preventive Interventions on the Early Risk Behaviors for Later Substance Abuse, Depression, and Antisocial Behavior." *American Journal of Community Psychology* 27 (5): 599–641.

IJzendoorn, M. H. van, J. Belsky, and M. J. Bakermans-Kranenburg. 2012. "Serotonin Transporter Genotype 5HTTLPR as a Marker of Differential Susceptibility? A Meta-Analysis of Child and Adolescent Gene-by-Environment Studies." *Translational Psychiatry* 2: e147.

Isometsä, E. T., and J. K. Lönnqvist. 1998. "Suicide Attempts Preceding Completed Suicide." *British Journal of Psychiatry* 173 (6): 531–35.

Ivison, K. 2011. *Red One: A Bomb Disposal Expert on the Front Line.* London: Phoenix.

Jablensky, A. 2009. "Epidemiology of Schizophrenia." In *New Oxford Textbook of Psychiatry*, 2nd ed., edited by M. G. Gelder, N. C. Andreasen, J. J. Lopez-Ibor Jr., and J. R. Geddes, 540–52. Oxford: Oxford University Press.

Jacobs, T. L., E. S. Epel, J. Lin, E. H. Blackburn, O. M. Wolkowitz, D. A. Bridwell, . . . C. D. Saron. 2011. "Intensive Meditation Training, Immune Cell Telomerase Activity, and Psychological Mediators." *Psychoneuroendocrinology* 36 (5): 664–81.

James, D. J., and L. E. Glaze. 2006. *Mental Health Problems of Prison and Jail Inmates.* Bureau of Justice Statistics, September.

James, O. 2007. *Affluenza: How to Be Successful and Stay Sane.* London: Vermilion.

————. 2008. *The Selfish Capitalist: Origins of Affluenza.* London: Vermilion.

Jones, S., L. Howard, and G. Thornicroft. 2008. "'Diagnostic Overshadowing': Worse Physical Health Care for People with Mental Illness." *Acta Psychiatrica Scandinavica* 118 (3): 169–71.

Judd, L. L., H. S. Akiskal, P. J. Schettler, J. Endicott, J. Maser, D. A. Solomon, . . . M. B. Keller. 2002. "The Long-Term Natural History of the Weekly Symptomatic Status of Bipolar I Disorder." *Archives of General Psychiatry* 59 (6): 530–37.

Kahneman, D. 2011. *Thinking, Fast and Slow.* London: Allen Lane.

Kanavos, P., S. van den Aardweg, and W. Schurer. 2012. *Diabetes Expenditure, Burden of Disease, and Management in 5 EU Countries.* London: LSE Health, London School of Economics and Political Science.

Karlin, B. E., G. K. Brown, M. Trockel, D. Cunning, A. M. Zeiss, and C. M. Taylor. 2012. "National Dissemination of Cognitive Behavioral Therapy for Depression in the Department of Veterans Affairs Health Care System: Therapist and Patient-Level Outcomes." *Journal of Consulting and Clinical Psychology* 80 (5): 707–18.

Karlin, B. E., and G. Cross. 2014. "From the Laboratory to the Therapy Room: National Dissemination and Implementation of Evidence-Based Psychotherapies in the US Department of Veterans Affairs Health Care System." *American Psychologist* 69: 19–33.

Karlin, B. E., J. F. Ruzek, C. M. Chard, A. Eftekhari, C. M. Monson, E. A. Hembree, P. A. Resick, and E. B. Foa. 2010. "Dissemination of Evidence-Based Psychological Treatments for Posttraumatic Stress Disorder in the Veterans Health Administration." *Journal of Traumatic Stress* 23 (6): 663–73.

Karlin, B. E., M. Trockel, C. B. Taylor, J. Gimeno, and R. Manber. 2013. "National Dissemination of Cognitive Behavioral Therapy for Insomnia in Veterans: Therapist and Patient-Level

Outcomes." *Journal of Consulting and Clinical Psychology* 81 (5): 912–17.

Kataoka, S. H., L. Zhang, and K. B. Wells. 2002. "Unmet Need for Mental Health Care among U.S. Children: Variation by Ethnicity and Insurance Status." *American Journal of Psychiatry* 159 (9): 1548–55.

Katon, W. J. 2003. "Clinical and Health Services Relationships between Major Depression, Depressive Symptoms, and General Medical Illness." *Society of Biological Psychiatry* 54: 216–26.

Katzelnick, D. J., K. A. Kobak, T. DeLeire, H. J. Henk, J. H. Greist, J.R.T. Davidson, . . . C. P. Helstad. 2001. "Impact of Generalized Social Anxiety Disorder in Managed Care." *American Journal of Psychiatry* 158: 1999–2007.

Kazdin, A. E. 2009. *The Kazdin Method for Parenting the Defiant Child: With No Pills, No Therapy, No Contest of Wills.* New York: First Mariner Books.

Kellam, S. G., C. H. Brown, J. M. Poduska, N. S. Ialongo, W. Wang, P. Toyinbo, . . . H. C. Wilcox. 2008. "Effects of a Universal Classroom Behavior Management Program in First and Second Grades on Young Adult Behavioral, Psychiatric, and Social Outcomes." *Drug and Alcohol Dependence* 95S: S5–S28.

Kelly, B., J. Longbottom, F. Potts, and J. Williamson. 2004. "Applying Emotional Intelligence: Exploring the Promoting Alternative Thinking Strategies Curriculum." *Educational Psychology in Practice* 20 (3): 221–40.

Kelvin, R., R. Layard, and A. York. 2009. "Improving Tier 2–3 CAMHS." *LSE CEP mimeo.*

Kendler, K. S., R. C. Kessler, E. E. Walters, C. MacLean, M. C. Neale, A. C. Health, and L. J. Eaves. 1995. "Stressful Life Events, Genetic Liability, and Onset of an Episode of Major Depression in Women." *American Journal of Psychiatry* 152 (6): 833–42.

Kendler, K. S., M. C. Neale, R. C. Kessler, A. C. Heath, and L. J. Eaves. 1992. "Major Depression and Generalized Anxiety

Disorder: Same Genes, (Partly) Different Environments?" *Archives of General Psychiatry* 49: 716–22.

Kendler, K. S., C. A. Prescott, J. Myers, and M. C. Neale. 2003. "The Structure of Genetic and Environmental Risk Factors for Common Psychiatric and Substance Use Disorders in Men and Women." *Archives of General Psychiatry* 60: 929–37.

Kennedy, I. 2010. *Getting It Right for Children and Young People: Overcoming Cultural Barriers in the NHS So as to Meet Their Needs.* A review by Professor Sir Ian Kennedy. London: Department of Health.

Kessler, R. C., P. Berglund, O. Demler, R. Jin, k. R. Merikangas, and E. E. Walters. 2005a. "Lifetime Prevalence and Age-of-Onset Distributions of DSM-IV Disorders in the National Comorbidity Survey Replication." *Archives of General Psychiatry* 62: 593–602.

Kessler, R. C., W. T. Chiu, O. Demler, K. R. Merikangas, and E. E. Walters. 2005b. "Prevalence, Severity, and Comorbidity of 12-Month DSM-IV Disorders in the National Comorbidity Survey Replication." *Archives of General Psychiatry* 62 (6): 617–27.

Kessler, R. C., O. Demler, R. G. Frank, M. Olfson, H. A. Pincus, E. E. Walters, . . . A. M. Zaslavsky. 2005c. "Prevalence and Treatment of Mental Disorders, 1990 to 2003." *New England Journal of Medicine* 352 (24): 2515–23.

Kessler, R. C., K. A. McGonagle, C. B. Nelson, M. Hughes, M. Swartz, and D. G. Blazer. 1994. "Sex and Depression in the National Comorbidity Survey, II: Cohort Effects." *Journal of Affective Disorders* 30: 15–26.

Kessler, R., and T. B. Üstün, eds. 2008. *The WHO World Mental Health Surveys: Global Perspectives on the Epidemiology of Mental Disorders.* New York: Cambridge University Press.

Kety, S. S., P. H. Wender, B. Jacobsen, L. J. Ingraham, L. Janson, B. Faber, and D. K. Kinney. 1994. "Mental Illness in the Biological and Adoptive Relatives of Schizophrenic Adoptees:

Replication of the Copenhagen Study in the Rest of Denmark." *Archives of General Psychiatry* 51 (6): 442–55.

Kiecolt-Glaser, J. K., P. T. Marucha, W. B. Malarkey, A. M. Mercado, and R. Glaser. 1995. "Slowing of Wound Healing by Psychological Stress." *Lancet* 346: 1194–96.

Kiecolt-Glaser, J. K., L. McGuire, T. F. Robles, and R. Glaser. 2002. "Emotions, Morbidity, and Mortality: New Perspectives from Psychoneuroimmunology." *Annual Review of Psychology* 53: 83–107.

Kieling, C., H. Baker-Henningham, M. Belfer, G. Conti, I. Ertem, O. Omigbodun, . . . A. Rahman. 2011. "Child and Adolescent Mental Health Worldwide: Evidence for Action." *Lancet* 378: 1515–25.

Kim-Cohen, J., A. Caspi, T. E. Moffitt, H. Harrington, B. J. Milne, and R. Poulton. 2003. "Prior Juvenile Diagnoses in Adults with Mental Disorder: Developmental Follow-Back of a Prospective-Longitudinal Cohort." *Archives of General Psychiatry* 60: 709–17.

Kirkbride, J. B., A. Errazuriz, T. J. Croudace, C. Morgan, D. Jackson, J. Boydell, . . . P. B. Jones. 2012. "Incidence of Schizophrenia and Other Psychoses in England, 1950–2009: A Systematic Review and Meta-Analyses." *PLoS ONE* 7 (3): e31660.

Knapp, M., D. McDaid, and M. Parsonage, eds. 2011. *Mental Health Promotion and Mental Illness Prevention: The Economic Case*. London: Department of Health.

Knies, G. 2012. "Life Satisfaction and Material Well-Being of Children in the UK." ISER Working Paper Series No. 2012–15. University of Essex: Institute for Social and Economic Research.

Kocsis, J. H., A. C. Leon, J. C. Markowitz, R. Manber, B. Arnow, D. N. Klein, and M. E. Thase. 2009. "Patient Preference as a Moderator of Outcome for Chronic Forms of Major Depressive Disorder Treated with Nefazodone, Cognitive Behavioural Analysis System of Psychotherapy, or Their Combination." *Journal of Clinical Psychiatry* 70 (3): 354–61.

Kopelowicz, A., R. P. Liberman, and R. Zarate. 2007. "Psychosocial

Treatments for Schizophrenia." In *A Guide to Treatments That Work*, 3rd ed., edited by P. E. Nathan and J. M. Gorman. New York: Oxford University Press.

Kroenke, K., R. L. Spitzer, and J.B.W. Williams. 2001. "The PHQ-9: Validity of a Brief Depression Severity Measure." *Journal of General Internal Medicine* 16: 606–13.

Kross, E., M. G. Berman, W. Mischel, E. E. Smith, and T. D. Wager. 2011. "Social Rejection Shares Somatosensory Representations with Physical Pain." *Proceedings of the National Academy of Sciences (PNAS)* 108 (15): 6270–75.

Kumari, M., M. Shipley, M. Stafford, and M. Kivimaki. 2011. "Association of Diurnal Patterns in Salivary Cortisol with All-Cause and Cardiovascular Mortality: Findings from the Whitehall II Study." *Journal of Clinical Endocrinology and Metabolism* 96 (5): 1478–85.

Ladapo, J. A., J. A. Shaffer, Y. Fang, S. Ye, and K. W. Davidson. 2012. "Cost-Effectiveness of Enhanced Depression Care after Acute Coronary Syndrome: Results from the Coronary Psychosocial Evaluation Studies Randomized Controlled Trial." *Archives of Internal Medicine* 172 (21): 1682–83.

Lagerveld, S. E., R.W.B. Blonk, V. Brenninkmeijer, L. Wijngaards-de Meij, and W. B. Schaufeli. 2012. "Work-Focused Treatment of Common Mental Disorders and Return to Work: A Comparative Outcome Study." *Journal of Occupational Health Psychology* 17 (2): 220–34.

Layard, R. 2005. "Mental Health: Britain's Biggest Social Problem?" No. 10 Strategy Unit Seminar on Mental Health. *LSE CEP mimeo*.

———. 2009. "The Greatest Happiness Principle: Its Time Has Come." In *Well-Being: How to Lead the Good Life and What Government Should Do To Help*, edited by S. Griffiths and R. Reeves, 92–106. London: Social Market Foundation.

———. 2011a. *Happiness: Lessons from a New Science*. 2nd ed. London: Penguin.

———. 2011b. "Well-Being and Action for Happiness." In *Changing the Debate: The Ideas Redefining Britain*, 22–26. London: ResPublica.

Layard, R., D. Chisholm, V. Patel, and S. Saxena. 2013a. "Mental Illness and Unhappiness." In *World Happiness Report 2013*, edited by J. F. Helliwell, R. Layard, and J. Sachs, 38–53. New York: Sustainable Development Solutions Network.

Layard, R., A. E. Clark, F. Cornaglia, N. Powdthavee, and J. Vernoit. 2013b. "What Predicts a Successful Life? A Life-Course Model of Well-Being." CEP Discussion Paper No. 1245. London: LSE Centre for Economic Performance.

Layard, R., A. E. Clark, and C. Senik. 2012. "The Causes of Happiness and Misery." In *World Happiness Report*, edited by J. F. Helliwell, R. Layard, and J. Sachs, 58–89. New York: Earth Institute, Columbia University.

Layard, R., D. M. Clark, M. Knapp, and G. Mayraz. 2007. "Cost-Benefit Analysis of Psychological Therapy." *National Institute Economic Review* 202: 90–98.

Layard, R., and J. Dunn. 2009. *A Good Childhood: Searching for Values in a Competitive Age*. Report for the Children's Society. London: Penguin.

Layard, R., and A. Hagell. 2015. *Healthy Young Minds: Transforming the Mental Health of Children*. Report of the Mental Health and Wellbeing in Children Forum to the World Innovation Summit for Health (WISH) 2015. Reprinted in World Happiness Report 2015, edited by J. F. Helliwell, R. Layard, and J. Sachs. New York: UN Sustainable Development Solutions Network.

Layard, R., G. Mayraz, and S. J. Nickell. 2010. "Does Relative Income Matter? Are the Critics Right?" In *International Differences in Well-Being*, edited by E. Diener, J. F. Helliwell, and D. Kahneman, 139–65. New York: Oxford University Press.

Layard, R., S. J. Nickell, and G. Mayraz. 2008. "The Marginal Utility of Income." *Journal of Public Economics, Special Issue: Happiness and Public Economics* 92 (8–9): 1846–57.

Lee, S., S. Aos, E. Drake, A. Pennucci, M. Miller, and L. Anderson. 2012. *Return on Investment: Evidence-Based Options to Improve Statewide Outcomes.* Document No. 12-04-1201. Olympia: Washington State Institute for Public Policy.

Leff, J., L. Kuipers, R. Berkowitz, R. Eberlein-Fries, and D. Sturgeon. 1982. "A Controlled Trial of Social Intervention in Families of Schizophrenic Patients." *British Journal of Psychiatry* 141: 121–34.

Leichsenring, F., S. Salzer, M. E. Beutel, S. Herpertz, W. Hiller, J. Hoyer, . . . E. Leibing. 2013. "Psychodynamic Therapy and Cognitive Behavioral Therapy in Social Anxiety Disorder: A Multicenter Randomized Controlled Trial." *American Journal of Psychiatry* 170 (7): 759–67.

Leveson, B. 2012. *An Inquiry into the Culture, Practices, and Ethics of the Press.* London: The Stationery Office (TSO).

Levit, K. R., T. L. Mark, R. M. Coffey, S. Frankel, P. Santora, R. Vandivort-Warren, and K. Malone. 2013. "Federal Spending On Behavioral Health Accelerated During Recession As Individuals Lost Employer Insurance." *Health Affairs* 32 (5): 952–62.

Lewin, B., I. H. Robertson, E. L. Cay, J. B. Irving, and M. Campbell. 1992. "Effects of Self-Help Post-Myocardial-Infarction Rehabilitation on Psychological Adjustment and Use of Health Services." *Lancet* 339 (8800): 1036–40.

Lincoln, T. M., W. Rief, K. Hahlweg, M. Frank, I. von Witzleben, B. Schroeder, and W. Fiegenbaum. 2003. "Effectiveness of an Empirically Supported Treatment for Social Phobia in the Field." *Behaviour Research and Therapy* 41 (11): 1251–69.

Linehan, M. M., K. A. Comtois, A. M. Murray, M. Z. Brown, R. J. Gallop, H. L. Heard, . . . N. Lindenboim. 2006. "Two-Year Randomized Controlled Trial and Follow-Up of Dialectical Behaviour Therapy vs Therapy by Experts for Suicidal

Behaviours and Borderline Personality Disorder." *Archives of General Psychiatry* 63: 757–66.

Little, M., V. Berry, L. Morpeth, S. Blower, N. Axford, R. Taylor, . . . K. Tobin. 2012. "The Impact of Three Evidence-Based Programmes Delivered in Public Systems in Birmingham, UK." *International Journal of Conflict and Violence* 6 (2): 260–72.

Lochman, J., K. C. Wells, and L. A. Lenhart. 2008. *Coping Power: Child Group Program (Facilitator Guide)*. Oxford: Oxford University Press.

Lorberbaum, J. P., J. D. Newman, J. R. Dubno, A. R. Horwitz, Z. Nahas, C. C. Teneback, . . . M. S. George. 1999. "Feasibility of Using fMRI to Study Mothers Responding to Infant Cries." *Depression and Anxiety* 10: 99–104.

Löwe, B., O. Decker, S. Müller, E. Brähler, D. Schellberg, W. Herzog, and P. Y. Herzberg. 2008. "Validation and Standardization of the Generalized Anxiety Disorder Screener (GAD-7) in the General Population." *Medical Care* 46 (3): 266–74.

LSE Centre for Economic Performance's Mental Health Policy Group. 2006. *The Depression Report: A New Deal for Depression and Anxiety Disorders*. London: London School of Economics and Political Science.

———. 2012. *How Mental Illness Loses Out in the NHS*. London: London School of Economics and Political Science.

Lucas, R. E. 2003. "Macroeconomic Priorities." *American Economic Review* 93 (1): 1–14.

Lucas, R. E., A. E. Clark, Y. Georgellis, and E. Diener. 2004. "Unemployment Alters the Set Point for Life Satisfaction." *Psychological Science* 15 (1): 8–13.

Lund, C., M. De Silva, S. Plagerson, S. Cooper, D. Chisholm, J. Das, . . . V. Patel. 2011. "Poverty and Mental Disorders: Breaking the Cycle in Low-Income and Middle-Income Countries." *Lancet* 378 (9801): 1502–14.

Lundberg, U., and C. L. Cooper. 2011. *The Science of Occupational*

Health: Stress, Psychobiology, and the New World of Work. Oxford: Wiley-Blackwell.

Lundborg, P., A. Nilsson, and D.-O. Rooth. 2011. "Early Life Health and Adult Earnings: Evidence from a Large Sample of Siblings and Twins." IZA Discussion Paper No. 5804.

Mansell, W., D. M. Clark, and A. Ehlers. 2003. "Internal versus External Attention in Social Anxiety: An Investigation Using a Novel Paradigm." *Behaviour Research and Therapy* 41 (5): 555–72.

Manson, J. E., J. Hsia, K. C. Johnson, J. E. Rossouw, A. R. Assaf, N. L. Lasser, . . . M. Cushman for the Women's Health Initiative Investigators. 2003. "Estrogen Plus Progestin and the Risk of Coronary Heart Disease." *New England Journal of Medicine* 349: 523–34.

Marmot, M., J. Allen, P. Goldblatt, T. Boyce, D. McNeish, M. Grady, and I. Geddes. 2010. *Fair Society, Healthy Lives—The Marmot Review: Strategic Review of Health Inequalities in England Post-2010.* London: Marmot Review.

Marmot, M., I. Gilmore, A. Britton, R. Doll, G. Edwards, C. Godfrey, . . . R. Room. 2004. *Calling Time: The Nation's Drinking as a Major Health Issue.* London: Academy of Medical Sciences.

Martin, A., W. Rief, A. Klaiberg, and E. Braehler. 2006. "Validity of the Brief Patient Health Questionnaire Mood Scale (PHQ-9) in the General Population." *General Hospital Psychiatry* 28: 71–77.

Mattson, S. N., N. Crocker, and T. T. Nguyen. 2011. "Fetal Alcohol Spectrum Disorders: Neuropsychological and Behavioral Features." *Neuropsychology Review* 21: 81–101.

Maughan, B., S. Collishaw, H. Meltzer, and R. Goodman. 2008. "Recent Trends in UK Child and Adolescent Mental Health." *Social Psychiatry and Psychiatric Epidemiology* 43: 305–10.

Mayo-Wilson, E., S. Dias, I. Mavranezouli, K. Kew, D. M. Clark, A. Ades, and S. Pilling. 2014. "Psychological and Pharmacological Interventions for Social Anxiety Disorder in Adults: A

Systematic Review and Network Meta-Analysis." *Lancet Psychiatry* 1: 368–76.

Mayou, R. A., A. Ehlers, and M. Hobbs. 2000. "Psychological Debriefing for Road Traffic Accident Victims: Three-Year Follow-Up of a Randomised Controlled Trial." *British Journal of Psychiatry* 176 (6): 589–93.

McCrone, P., M. Knapp, J. Proudfoot, C. Ryden, K. Cavanagh, D. A. Shapiro, . . . A. Tylee. 2004. "Cost-Effectiveness of Computerised Cognitive Behavioural Therapy for Anxiety and Depression in Primary Care: Randomised Controlled Trial." *British Journal of Psychiatry* 185: 55–62.

McDaid, D., and A.-L. Park. 2011. "Investing in Mental Health and Well-Being: Findings from the DataPrev Project." *Health Promotion International* 26 (S1): i108–39.

McEwen, B. S. 1998. "Protective and Damaging Effects of Stress Mediators." *New England Journal of Medicine* 338 (3): 171–79.

McGuffin, P., M. J. Owen, and I. I. Gottesman, eds. 2004. *Psychiatric Genetics and Genomics*. Oxford: Oxford University Press.

McHugh, R. K., S. W. Whitton, A. D. Peckham, J. A. Welge, and M. W. Otto. 2013. "Patient Preference for Psychological versus Pharmacologic Treatment of Psychiatric Disorders: A Meta-Analytic Review." *Journal of Clinical Psychiatry* 74 (6): 595–602.

McManus, S., H. Meltzer, T. Brugha, P. Bebbington, and R. Jenkins, eds. 2009. *Adult Psychiatric Morbidity in England, 2007: Results of a Household Survey*. Leeds: Health and Social Care Information Centre, Social Care Statistics.

Meade, B., and B. Steiner. 2010. "The Total Effects of Boot Camps That House Juveniles: A Systematic Review of the Evidence." *Journal of Criminal Justice* 38: 841–53.

Melhuish, E., J. Belsky, A. H. Leyland, J. Barnes, and the National Evaluation of Sure Start Research Team. 2008. "Effects of Fully-Established Sure Start Local Programmes on 3-Year-Old Children and Their Families Living in England: A Quasi-Experimental Observational Study." *Lancet* 372: 1641–47.

Meltzer, H., R. Gatward, T. Corbin, R. Goodman, and T. Ford. 2003. *Persistence, Onset, Risk Factors, and Outcomes of Childhood Mental Disorders*. Office for National Statistics (ONS). London: The Stationery Office (TSO).

Meltzer, H., B. Gill, M. Petticrew, and K. Hinds. 1995. *OPCS Surveys of Psychiatric Morbidity in Great Britain, Report 1: The Prevalence of Psychiatric Morbidity among Adults Living in Private Households*. London: HMSO.

Merikangas, K. R., R. Jin, J. P. He, R. C. Kessler, S. Lee, N. A. Sampson, . . . Z. Zarkov. 2011. "Prevalence and Correlates of Bipolar Spectrum Disorder in the World Mental Health Survey Initiative." *Archives of General Psychiatry* 68 (3): 241–51.

Merrill, K. A., V. E. Tolbert, and W. A. Wade. 2003. "Effectiveness of Cognitive Therapy for Depression in a Community Mental Health Center: A Benchmarking Study." *Journal of Consulting and Clinical Psychology* 71 (2): 404–9.

Moffitt, T. E. 1993. "Adolescence-Limited and Life-Course-Persistent Antisocial Behavior: A Developmental Taxonomy." *Psychological Review* 100 (4): 674–701.

———. 2003. "Life-Course-Persistent and Adolescence-Limited Antisocial Behavior: A 10-Year Research Review and a Research Agenda." In *Causes of Conduct Disorder and Juvenile Delinquency*, edited by B. B. Lahey, T. E. Moffitt, and A. Caspi, 49–75. New York: Guilford Press.

Molosankwe, I., A. Patel, J. J. Gagliardino, M. Knapp, and D. McDaid. 2012. "Economic Aspects of the Association between Diabetes and Depression: A Systematic Review." *Journal of Affective Disorders* 142S (1): S42–S55.

Monroe, S. M., and K. L. Harkness. 2011. "Recurrence in Major Depression: A Conceptual Analysis." *Psychological Review* 118 (4): 655–74.

Moore, R.K.G., D. G. Groves, J. D. Bridson, A. D. Grayson, H. Wong, A. Leach, . . . M. R. Chester. 2007. "A Brief Cognitive Behavioral Intervention Reduces Hospital Admissions in

Refractory Angina Patients," *Journal of Pain and Symptom Management* 33 (3): 310–16.

Morens, D. M. 1999. "Death of a President." *New England Journal of Medicine* 341 (24): 1845–49.

Mörtberg, E., D. M. Clark, and S. Bejerot. 2011. "Intensive Group Cognitive Therapy and Individual Cognitive Therapy for Social Phobia: Sustained Improvement at 5-Year Follow-Up." *Journal of Anxiety Disorders* 25 (8): 994–1000.

Moses, H., D.H.M. Matheson, S. Cairns-Smith, B. P. George, C. Palisch, and E. R. Dorsey. 2015. "The Anatomy of Medical Research: US and International Comparisons." *JAMA* 313 (2): 174–89.

Moussavi, S., S. Chatterji, E. Verdes, A. Tandon, V. Patel, and B. Ustun. 2007. "Depression, Chronic Diseases, and Decrements in Health: Results from the World Health Surveys." *Lancet* 370 (9590): 851–58.

Mykletun, A., O. Bjerkeset, S. Overland, M. Prince, M. Dewey, and R. Stewart. 2009. "Levels of Anxiety and Depression as Predictors of Mortality: The HUNT Study." *British Journal of Psychiatry* 195: 118–25.

Naipaul, S. 1985. *Beyond the Dragon's Mouth*. London: Abacus.

National Confidential Inquiry into Suicide and Homicide by People with Mental Illness (NCISH). 2013. *Annual Report: England, Northern Ireland, Scotland, and Wales*. Commissioned by the Healthcare Quality Improvement Partnership (HQIP). Manchester: Centre for Mental Health and Risk, University of Manchester.

National Family and Parenting Institute (NFPI). 2000. *Teenagers' Attitudes to Parenting: A Survey of Young People's Experiences of Being Parented, and Their Views on How to Bring Up Children*. NFPI survey conducted by MORI. London: National Family and Parenting Institute.

Naylor, C., M. Parsonage, D. McDaid, M. Knapp, M. Fossey, and A. Galea. 2012. *Long-Term Conditions and Mental Health: The*

Cost of Co-Morbidities. London: King's Fund and Centre for Mental Health.

Neill, S. 2008. *Disruptive Pupil Behaviour: Its Causes and Effects (A Survey Analysed for the National Union of Teachers).* London: National Union of Teachers.

NHS Confederation. 2012. *Investing in Emotional and Psychological Wellbeing for Patients with Long-Term Conditions.* London: NHS Confederation Mental Health Network.

NICE. 2004. *Eating Disorders: Core Interventions in the Treatment and Management of Anorexia Nervosa, Bulimia Nervosa, and Related Eating Disorders (Clinical Guideline 9).* London: National Institute for Clinical Excellence.

————. 2005a. *Depression in Children and Young People: Identification and Management in Primary, Community, and Secondary Care (Clinical Guideline 28).* London: National Institute for Health and Clinical Excellence.

————. 2005b. *Obsessive-Compulsive Disorder: Core Interventions in the Treatment of Obsessive-Compulsive Disorder and Body Dysmorphic Disorder (Clinical Guideline 31).* London: National Institute for Health and Clinical Excellence.

————. 2005c. *Post-Traumatic Stress Disorder (PTSD): The Management of PTSD in Adults and Children in Primary and Secondary Care (Clinical Guideline 26).* London: National Institute for Clinical Excellence.

————. 2007. *Drug Misuse: Psychosocial Interventions (Clinical Guideline 51).* London: National Institute for Health and Clinical Excellence.

————. 2009a. *Borderline Personality Disorder: Treatment and Management (Clinical Guideline 78).* London: National Institute of Health and Clinical Excellence.

————. 2009b. *Depression in Adults with a Chronic Physical Problem: Treatment and Management (Clinical Guideline 91).* London: National Institute for Health and Care Excellence.

————. 2009c. *Depression in Adults: The Treatment and Management of Depression in Adults (Clinical Guideline 90).* London: National Institute of Health and Clinical Excellence.

————. 2009d. *Schizophrenia: Core Interventions in the Treatment and Management of Schizophrenia in Adults in Primary and Secondary Care (Clinical Guideline 82).* London: National Institute for Health and Clinical Excellence.

————. 2011a. *Alcohol-Use Disorders: Diagnosis, Assessment, and Management of Harmful Drinking and Alcohol Dependence (Clinical Guideline 115).* London: National Institute of Health and Clinical Excellence.

————. 2011b. *Autism Diagnosis in Children and Young People: Recognition, Referral, and Diagnosis of Children and Young People on the Autism Spectrum (Clinical Guideline 128).* London: National Institute for Health and Clinical Excellence.

————. 2011c. *Generalised Anxiety Disorder and Panic Disorder (with or without Agoraphobia) in Adults: Management in Primary, Secondary, and Community Care (Clinical Guideline 113).* London: National Institute for Health and Clinical Excellence.

————. 2013a. *Antisocial Behaviour and Conduct Disorders in Children and Young People: Recognition, Intervention, and Management (Clinical Guideline 158).* London: National Institute for Health and Care Excellence.

————. 2013b. *Antisocial Personality Disorder: Treatment, Management, and Prevention (Clinical Guideline 77).* London: National Institute of Health and Clinical Excellence.

————. 2013c. *Attention Deficit Hyperactivity Disorder: Diagnosis and Management of ADHD in Children, Young People and Adults (Clinical Guideline 72).* London: National Institute for Health and Clinical Excellence.

————. 2013d. *Social Anxiety Disorder: Recognition, Assessment, and Treatment (Clinical Guideline 159).* London: National Institute for Health and Care Excellence.

Nicholson, A., H. Kuper, and H. Hemingway. 2006. "Depression as an Aetiologic and Prognostic Factor in Coronary Heart Disease: A Meta-Analysis of 6,362 Events among 146,538 Participants in 54 Observational Studies." *European Heart Journal* 27: 2763–74.

Nimnuan, C., M. Hotopf, and S. Wessely. 2001. "Medically Unexplained Symptoms: An Epidemiological Study in Seven Specialties." *Journal of Psychosomatic Research* 51 (1): 361–67.

Nutt, D. 2012. *Drugs—Without the Hot Air: Minimising the Harms of Legal and Illegal Drugs*. Cambridge: UIT Cambridge.

O'Donnell, G., A. Deaton, M. Durand, D. Halpern, and R. Layard. 2014. *Wellbeing and Policy*. London: Legatum Institute.

OECD. 2012. *Sick on the Job? Myths and Realities about Mental Health and Work*. Paris: OECD Publishing.

———. 2013. *OECD Guidelines on Measuring Subjective Well-Being*. Paris: OECD Publishing.

Ofsted. 2013. *Not Yet Good Enough: Personal, Social, Health and Economic Education in Schools*. Manchester: Office for Standards in Education, Children's Services and Skills (Ofsted).

Olds, D., C. R. Henderson, R. Cole, J. Eckenrode, H. Kitzman, D. Luckey, . . . J. Powers. 1998. "Long-Term Effects of Nurse Home Visitation on Children's Criminal and Antisocial Behavior: 15-Year Follow-Up of a Randomized Controlled Trial." *JAMA* 280 (14): 1238–44.

Ormel, J., M. Petukhova, S. Chatterji, S. Aguilar-Gaxiola, J. Alonso, M. C. Angermeyer, . . . R. C. Kessler. 2008. "Disability and Treatment of Specific Mental and Physical Disorders across the World." *British Journal of Psychiatry* 192: 368–75.

Ost, L. G. 2009. Long-Term Results of CBT in Anxiety Disorders.

Ost, L. G., J. Fellenius, and U. Sterner. 1991. "Applied Tension, Exposure in vivo, and Tension Only in the Treatment of Blood Phobia." *Behaviour Research and Therapy* 29 (6): 561–75.

Pan, A., Q. Sun, O. I. Okereke, K. M. Rexrode, and F. B. Hu.

2011. "Depression and Risk of Stroke Morbidity and Mortality: A Meta-Analysis and Systematic Review." *JAMA* 306 (11): 1241–49.

Parks, G. 2000. *The High/Scope Perry Preschool Project.* Office of Juvenile Justice and Delinquency Prevention. Washington, DC: US Department of Justice.

Parsonage, M., and M. Fossey. 2011. *Economic Evaluation of a Liaison Psychiatry Service.* London: Centre for Mental Health.

Patten, S. B., J.V.A. Williams, D. H. Lavorato, G. Modgill, N. Jetté, and M. Eliasziw. 2008. "Major Depression as a Risk Factor for Chronic Disease Incidence: Longitudinal Analyses in a General Population Cohort." *General Hospital Psychiatry* 30: 407–13.

Paul, G. L. 1966. *Insight vs. Desensitisation in Psychotherapy: An Experiment in Anxiety Reduction.* Stanford, CA: Stanford University Press.

Pauly, M. V., S. Nicholson, J. Xu, D. Polsky, P. M. Danzon, J. F. Murray, and M. L. Berger. 2002. "A General Model of the Impact of Absenteeism on Employers and Employees." *Health Economics* 11: 221–31.

Perou, R., R. H. Bitsko, S. J. Blumberg, P. Pastor, R. M. Ghandour, J. C. Gfroerer, . . . L. N. Huang. 2013. "Mental Health Surveillance among Children—United States, 2005–2011." *Morbidity and Mortality Weekly Report*: Centers for Disease Control and Prevention, 62: 1–35.

Pettitt, B., S. Greenhead, H. Khalifeh, V. Drennan, T. Hart, J. Hogg, . . . P. Moran. 2013. *At Risk, Yet Dismissed: The Criminal Victimisation of People with Mental Health Problems.* London: Victim Support.

Phillips, M. R., J. Zhang, Q. Shi, Z. Song, Z. Ding, S. Pang, . . . Z. Wang. 2009. "Prevalence, Treatment, and Associated Disability of Mental Disorders in Four Provinces in China during 2001–05: An Epidemiological Survey." *Lancet* 373: 2041–53.

Pimm, J., and M. Virathajenman. 2015. *Improving Recovery in Buckinghamshire: Plan, Do, Study, Act.* Paper presented at the

Psychological Therapies in the NHS Conference, London, September 11.

Pinker, S. 2002. *The Blank Slate*. London: Penguin.

———. 2011. *The Better Angels of Our Nature: The Decline of Violence in History and Its Causes*. London: Allen Lane.

Plomin, R., J. C. DeFries, V. S. Knopik, and J. M. Neiderhiser, eds. 2013. *Behavioral Genetics*. 6th ed. New York: Worth Publishers.

Polanczyk, G., M. S. de Lima, B. L. Horta, J. Biederman, and L. A. Rohde. 2007. "The Worldwide Prevalence of ADHD: A Systematic Review and Metaregression Analysis." *American Journal of Psychiatry* 164 (6): 942–48.

Prison Reform Trust. 2012. *Bromley Briefings Prison Factfile*. London: Prison Reform Trust.

President's New Freedom Commission on Mental Health. 2003. *Achieving the Promise: Transforming Mental Health Care in America*. Final Report. DHHS Pub. No. SMA-03-3832. Rockville, MD: U.S. Department of Health and Human Services.

Proudfoot, J., D. Guest, J. Carson, G. Dunn, and J. Gray. 1997. "Effect of Cognitive Behavioural Training on Job-Finding among Long-Term Unemployed People." *Lancet* 350: 96–100.

Raes, F., J. W. Griffith, K. Van der Gucht, and J.M.G. Williams. 2013. "School-Based Prevention and Reduction of Depression in Adolescents: A Cluster-Randomized Controlled Trial of a Mindfulness Group Program." *Mindfulness* (published online March 6, 2013).

Rai, D., P. Zitko, K. Jones, J. Lynch, and R. Araya. 2013. "Country- and Individual-Level Socioeconomic Determinants of Depression: Multilevel Cross-National Comparison." *British Journal of Psychiatry* 202: 195–203.

Regier, D. A., M. E. Farmer, D. S. Rae, B. Z. Locke, S. J. Keith, L. L. Judd, and F. K. Goodwin. 1990. "Comorbidity of Mental Disorders with Alcohol and Other Drug Abuse: Results from the Epidemiologic Catchment Area (ECA) Study." *JAMA* 264 (19): 2511–18.

Reinke, W. M., M. Stormont, C. Webster-Stratton, L. L. Newcomer, and K. C. Herman. 2012. "The Incredible Years Teacher Classroom Management Program: Using Coaching to Support Generalization to Real-World Classroom Settings." *Psychology in the Schools* 49 (5): 416–28.

Robertson, I., and C. L. Cooper. 2011. *Well-Being: Productivity and Happiness at Work*. London: Palgrave Macmillan.

Robinson, K. L., J. McBeth, and G. J. MacFarlane. 2004. "Psychological Distress and Premature Mortality in the General Population: A Prospective Study." *Annals of Epidemiology* 14: 467–72.

Roest, A. M., E. J. Martens, J. Denollet, and P. De Jonge. 2010. "Prognostic Association of Anxiety Post Myocardial Infarction with Mortality and New Cardiac Events: A Meta-Analysis." *Psychosomatic Medicine* 72: 563–69.

Rollman, B. L., B. H. Belnap, S. Mazumdar, P. R. Houck, F. Zhu, W. Gardner, . . . M. K. Shear. 2005. "A Randomized Trial to Improve the Quality of Treatment for Panic and Generalized Anxiety Disorders in Primary Care." *Archives of General Psychiatry* 62 (12): 1332–41.

Rose, S. C., J. Bisson, R. Churchill, and S. Wessely. 2002. "Psychological Debriefing for Preventing Post Traumatic Stress Disorder (PTSD)." *Cochrane Database of Systematic Reviews* (2): CD000560.

Roth, A., and P. Fonagy, eds. 2005. *What Works for Whom? A Critical Review of Psychotherapy Research*. 2nd ed. New York: Guilford Press.

Roth, A. D., and S. Pilling. 2008. "Using an Evidence-Based Methodology to Identify the Competences Required to Deliver Effective Cognitive and Behavioural Therapy for Depression and Anxiety Disorders." *Behavioural and Cognitive Psychotherapy* 36: 129–47.

Roy, A., and M. Linnoila. 1986. "Alcoholism and Suicide." *Suicide and Life-Threatening Behavior* 16 (2): 244–73.

Royal College of Psychiatrists. 2013. *Report of the Second Round of the National Audit of Psychological Therapies (NAPT) 2013*. London: Healthcare Quality Improvement Partnership.

Rush, A. J., A. T. Beck, M. Kovacs, and S. Hollon. 1977. "Comparative Efficacy of Cognitive Therapy and Pharmacotherapy in the Treatment of Depressed Outpatients." *Cognitive Therapy and Research* 1 (1): 17–37.

Russ, T. C., E. Stamatakis, M. Hamer, J. M. Starr, M. Kivimaki, and G. D. Batty. 2012. "Association between Psychological Distress and Mortality: Individual Participant Pooled Analysis of 10 Prospective Cohort Studies." *British Medical Journal* 345 (e4933).

Rutter, M. 2000. "Psychosocial Influences: Critiques, Findings, and Research Needs." *Development and Psychopathology* 12: 375–405.

———. 2004. "Intergenerational Continuities and Discontinuities in Psychological Problems." In *Human Development across Lives and Generations: The Potential for Change*, edited by P. L. Chase-Lansdale, K. Kiernan, and R. J. Friedman. New York and Cambridge: Cambridge University Press.

Rutter, M., D. Bishop, D. S. Pine, S. Scott, J. S. Stevenson, E. A. Taylor, and A. Thapar, eds. 2008. *Rutter's Child and Adolescent Psychiatry*. 5th ed. Oxford: Wiley-Blackwell.

Rutter, M., H. Giller, A. and Hagell. 1998. *Antisocial Behavior by Young People*. Cambridge: Cambridge University Press.

Rutz, W., L. von Knorring, and J. Walinder. 1992. "Long-Term Effects of an Educational Program for General Practitioners Given by the Swedish Committee for the Prevention and Treatment of Depression." *Acta Psychiatrica Scandinavica* 85 (1): 83–88.

Sainsbury Centre for Mental Health. 2007. *Mental Health at Work: Developing the Business Case*. Policy Paper 8. London: Sainsbury Centre for Mental Health.

———. 2009. *The Chance of a Lifetime: Preventing Early Conduct Problems and Reducing Crime*. London: Sainsbury Centre for Mental Health.

Sanders, M. R., C. Markie-Dadds, and K.M.T. Turner. 2003. *Theoretical, Scientific, and Clinical Foundations of the Triple P Positive*

Parenting Program: A Population Approach to the Promotion of Parenting Competence. Parenting Research and Practice Monograph No 1. Parenting and Family Support Centre, University of Queensland.

Satin, J. R., W. Linden, and M. J. Phillips. 2009. "Depression as a Predictor of Disease Progression and Mortality in Cancer Patients: A Meta-Analysis." *Cancer* 115: 5349–61.

Sawyer, M. G., S. Pfeiffer, S. H. Spence, L. Bond, B. Graetz, D. Kay,… J. Sheffield. 2010. "School-Based Prevention of Depression: A Randomised Controlled Study of the *beyondblue* Schools Research Initiative." *Journal of Child Psychology and Psychiatry* 51 (2): 199–209.

Saxena, S., G. Paraje, P. Sharan, G. Karam, and R. Sadana. 2006. "The 10/90 Divide in Mental Health Research: Trends over a 10-Year Period." *British Journal of Psychiatry* 188: 81–82.

Schonert-Reichl, K. A., and M. S. Lawlor. 2010. "The Effects of a Mindfulness-Based Education Program on Pre- and Early Adolescents' Well-Being and Social and Emotional Competence." *Mindfulness* 1: 137–51.

Scott, S., J. Briskman, and T. G. O'Connor. 2014. "Early Prevention of Antisocial Personality: Long-Term Follow-Up of Two Randomized Controlled Trials Comparing Indicated and Selective Approaches." *American Journal of Psychiatry* 171 (6): 649–57.

Scott, S., A. Carby, and A. Rendu. 2008. "Impact of Therapists' Skill on Effectiveness of Parenting Groups for Child Antisocial Behavior." *IoP mimeo*. London: King's College London, Institute of Psychiatry, and University College London.

Scott, S., M. Knapp, J. Henderson, and B. Maughan. 2001. "Financial Cost of Social Exclusion: Follow-Up Study of Antisocial Children into Adulthood." *British Medical Journal* 323 (7306): 1–5.

Scott, S., K. Sylva, M. Doolan, J. Price, B. Jacobs, C. Crook, and S. Landau. 2010. "Randomised Controlled Trial of Parent Groups for Child Antisocial Behaviour Targeting Multiple Risk Factors: The SPOKES Project." *Journal of Child Psychology and Psychiatry* 51 (1): 48–57.

Segal, Z. V., J.M.G. Williams, and J. D. Teasdale. 2013. *Mindfulness-Based Cognitive Therapy for Depression*. 2nd ed. New York: Guilford Press.

Seligman, M.E.P. 1992. *Helplessness: On Depression, Development, and Death*. New York: W. H. Freeman.

———. 2002. *Authentic Happiness: Using the New Positive Psychology to Realise Your Potential for Lasting Fulfillment*. New York: Free Press.

———. 2011. *Flourish: A Visionary New Understanding of Happiness and Well-Being*. New York: Free Press.

Sen, A. 2009. *The Idea of Justice*. London: Allen Lane.

Sennett, R. 2003. *Respect: The Formation of Character in a World of Inequality*. London: Allen Lane.

Seshamani, M., and A. Gray. 2004. "Time to Death and Health Expenditure: An Improved Model for the Impact of Demographic Change on Health Care Costs." *Age and Ageing* 33 (6): 556–61.

Sharpe, L., T. Sensky, N. Timberlake, B. Ryan, C. R. Brewin, and S. Allard. 2001. "A Blind, Randomized, Controlled Trial of Cognitive Behavioural Intervention for Patients with Recent Onset Rheumatoid Arthritis: Preventing Psychological and Physical Morbidity." *Pain* 89 (2–3): 275–83.

Shenk, J. W. 2006. *Lincoln's Melancholy: How Depression Challenged a President and Fueled His Greatness*. New York: Mariner Books.

Siev, J., and D. L. Chambless. 2007. "Specificity of Treatment Effects: Cognitive Therapy and Relaxation for Generalized Anxiety Disorder and Panic Disorders." *Journal of Consulting and Clinical Psychology* 75 (4): 513–22.

Sigvardsson, S., M. Bohman, and C. R. Cloninger. 1996. "Replication of Stockholm Adoption Study of Alcoholism: Confirmatory Cross-Fostering Analysis." *Archives of General Psychiatry* 53 (8): 681–87.

Simmons, P., C. J. Hawley, T. M. Gale, and T. Sivakumaran. 2010. "Service User, Patient, Client, User or Survivor: Describing Recipients of Mental Health Services." *Psychiatrist* 34: 20–23.

Simon, G. E., W. J. Katon, E.H.B. Lin, C. Rutter, W. G. Manning, M. von Korff, . . . B. A. Young. 2007. "Cost-Effectiveness of Systematic Depression Treatment among People with Diabetes Mellitus." *Archives of General Psychiatry* 64: 65–72.

Singer, T., B. Seymour, J. O'Doherty, H. Kaube, R. J. Dolan, and C. D. Frith. 2004. "Empathy for Pain Involves the Affective but Not Sensory Components of Pain." *Science* 303 (5661): 1157–62.

Singleton, N., R. Bumpstead, M. O'Brien, A. Lee, and H. Meltzer. 2001. *Psychiatric Morbidity among Adults Living in Private Households, 2000*. Office for National Statistics (ONS). London: The Stationery Office (TSO).

Singleton, N., and G. Lewis, eds. 2003. *Better or Worse: A Longitudinal Study of the Mental Health of Adults Living in Private Households in Great Britain*. Office for National Statistics (ONS). London: The Stationery Office.

Singleton, N., H. Meltzer, R. Gatward, with J. Coid and D. Deasy. 1998. *Psychiatric Morbidity among Prisoners in England and Wales*. Office for National Statistics (ONS). London: The Stationery Office (TSO).

Skidelsky, R., and E. Skidelsky. 2012. *How Much Is Enough? The Love of Money and the Case for the Good Life*. London: Allen Lane.

Smith, J. P., and G. C. Smith. 2010. "Long-Term Economic Costs of Psychological Problems during Childhood." *Social Science & Medicine* 71: 110–15.

Solomon, A. 2001. *The Noonday Demon: An Atlas of Depression*. London: Chatto and Windus.

Stallard, P., K. Sayal, T. Phillips, J. A. Taylor, M. Spears, R. Anderson, . . . A. A. Montgomery. 2012. "Classroom Based Cognitive Behavioural Therapy in Reducing Symptoms of Depression in

High Risk Adolescents: Pragmatic Cluster Randomised Controlled Trial." *British Medical Journal* 345 (7878): e6058.

Stangier, U., E. Schramm, T. Heidenreich, M. Berger, and D. M. Clark. 2011. "Cognitive Therapy vs Interpersonal Psychotherapy in Social Anxiety Disorder: A Randomized Controlled Trial." *Archives of General Psychiatry* 68 (7): 692–700.

Stanley, E. A., and A. P. Jha. 2009. "Mind Fitness: Improving Operational Effectiveness and Building Warrior Resilience." *Joint Force Quarterly* 55: 144–51.

Stein, M. B., J. R. McQuaid, C. Laffaye, and M. E. McCahill. 1999. "Social Phobia in the Primary Care Medical Setting." *Journal of Family Practice* 48 (7): 514–19.

Steptoe, A., and M. Kivimäki. 2012. "Stress and Cardiovascular Disease." *Nature Reviews Cardiology* 9: 360–70.

Steptoe, A., K. O'Donnell, E. Badrick, M. Kumari, and M. Marmot. 2008. "Neuroendocrine and Inflammatory Factors Associated with Positive Affect in Healthy Men and Women: The Whitehall II Study." *American Journal of Epidemiology* 167 (1): 96–102.

Steptoe, A., and J. Wardle. 2012. "Enjoying Life and Living Longer." *Archives of Internal Medicine* 172 (3): 273–75.

Steptoe, A., J. Wardle, and M. Marmot. 2005. "Positive Affect and Health-Related Neuroendocrine, Cardiovascular, and Inflammatory Processes." *Proceedings of the National Academy of Sciences (PNAS)* 102 (18): 6508–12.

Stevenson, B., and J. Wolfers. 2008. "Economic Growth and Subjective Well-Being: Reassessing the Easterlin Paradox." *Brookings Papers on Economic Activity* 2008 (1): 1–87.

———. 2010. "Inequality and Subjective Well-Being." Working paper.

Stiles, W. B., M. Barkham, J. Mellor-Clark, and J. Connell. 2008. "Effectiveness of Cognitive Behavioural, Person-Centred, and Psychodynamic Therapies in UK Primary-Care Routine Practice:

Replication in a Larger Sample." *Psychological Medicine* 38: 677–88.

Storr, A. 1990. *Churchill's Black Dog and Other Phenomena of the Human Mind.* London: Fontana.

Styron, W. 2001. *Darkness Visible: A Memoir of Madness.* London: Vintage.

Substance Abuse and Mental Health Services Administration (SAMHSA)—Center for Mental Health Services. 2007. *Promotion and Prevention in Mental Health: Strengthening Parenting and Enhancing Child Resilience.* US Department of Health and Human Services. Rockville, MD.

Sullivan, E. M., J. L. Annest, F. Luo, T. R. Simon, and L. L. Dahlberg. 2013. "Suicide among Adults Aged 35–64 Years: United States, 1999–2010." *Morbidity and Mortality Weekly Report (MMWR)* 62 (17): 321–25. US Department of Health and Human Services: Centers for Disease Control and Prevention.

Suomi, S. 1997. "Long-Term Effects of Different Early Rearing Experiences on Social, Emotional, and Physiological Development in Nonhuman Primates." In *Neurodevelopment and Adult Psychopathology*, edited by M. S. Keshavan and R. M. Murray. Cambridge: Cambridge University Press.

Teasdale, J. D., Z. V. Segal, J.M.G. Williams, V. Ridgeway, J. Soulsby, and M. Lau. 2000. "Prevention of Relapse/Recurrence in Major Depression by Mindfulness-Based Cognitive Therapy. *Journal of Consulting and Clinical Psychology* 68: 615–23.

Thornicroft, G. 2006. *Shunned: Discrimination against People with Mental Illness.* Oxford: Oxford University Press.

———. 2011. "Physical Health Disparities and Mental Illness: The Scandal of Premature Mortality." *British Journal of Psychiatry* 199: 441–42.

Timmins, N. 2001. *The Five Giants: A Biography of the Welfare State.* 2nd ed. London: HarperCollins.

Twenge, J. M., B. Gentile, C. N. DeWall, D. Ma, K. Lacefield, and D. R. Schurtz. 2010. "Birth Cohort Increases in Psychopathology among Young Americans, 1938–2007: A Cross-Temporal Meta-Analysis of the MMPI." *Clinical Psychology Review* 30: 145–54.

US Department of Health and Human Services. 2008. *Substance Abuse Prevention Dollars and Cents: A Cost-Benefit Analysis.* Substance Abuse and Mental Health Services Administration, Center for Substance Abuse Prevention.

Van Ameringen, M., C. Mancini, and P. Farvolden. 2003. "The Impact of Anxiety Disorders on Educational Achievement." *Journal of Anxiety Disorders* 17 (5): 561–71.

van Schaik, D.J.F., A.F.J. Klijn, H.P.J. van Hout, H.W.J. van Marwijk, A.T.F. Beekman, M. de Haan, and R. van Dyck. 2004. "Patients' Preferences in the Treatment of Depressive Disorder in Primary Care." *General Hospital Psychiatry* 26: 184–89.

Veale, D., and R. Willson, eds. 2011. *Taking Control of OCD: Inspirational Stories of Hope and Recovery.* London: Constable and Robinson.

Vos, T., A. D. Flaxman, M. Naghavi, R. Lozano, C. Michaud, M. Ezzati . . . C. J. L. Murray. 2012. "Years Lived with Disability (YLDs) for 1,160 Sequelae of 289 Diseases and Injuries, 1990–2010: A Systematic Analysis for the Global Burden of Disease Study 2010." *Lancet* 380: 2163–96.

Wampold, B. E., G. W. Mondin, M. Moody, F. Stich, K. Benson, and H. Ahn. 1997. "A Meta-Analysis of Outcome Studies Comparing Bona Fide Psychotherapies: Empirically, 'All Must Have Prizes.'" *Psychological Bulletin* 122 (3): 203–15.

Wang, P. S., P. Berglund, M. Olfson, H. A. Pincus, K. B. Wells, and R. C. Kessler. 2005. "Failure and Delay in Initial Treatment Contact after First Onset of Mental Disorders in the National Comorbidity Survey Replication." *Archives of General Psychiatry* 62: 603–13.

Weare, K. 2012. *Evidence for the Impact of Mindfulness on Children and Young People.* The Mindfulness in Schools Project.

Weare, K., and M. Nind. 2011. "Mental Health Promotion and

Problem Prevention in Schools: What Does the Evidence Say?" *Health Promotion International* 26 (S1): i29–i69.

Webster-Stratton, C., and M. J. Reid. 2010. "The Incredible Years Parents, Teachers, and Children Training Series: A Multifaceted Treatment Approach for Young Children with Conduct Disorders." In *Evidence-Based Psychotherapies for Children and Adolescents*, 2nd ed., edited by J. Weisz and A. Kazdin, 194–210. New York: Guilford Publications.

Webster-Stratton, C., M. J. Reid, and M. Hammond. 2001. "Preventing Conduct Problems, Promoting Social Competence: A Parent and Teacher Training Partnership in Head Start." *Journal of Clinical Child Psychology* 30 (3): 283–302.

Webster-Stratton, C., W. M. Reinke, K. C. Herman, and L. L. Newcomer. 2011. "The Incredible Years Teacher Classroom Management Training: The Methods and Principles That Support Fidelity of Training Delivery." *School Psychology Review* 40 (4): 509–29.

Weiss, B., A. Caron, S. Ball, J. Tapp, M. Johnson, and J. Weisz. 2005. "Iatrogenic Effects of Group Treatment for Antisocial Youth." *Journal of Consulting and Clinical Psychology* 73 (6): 1036–44.

Welch, C. A., D. Czerwinski, B. Ghimire, and D. Bertsimas. 2009. "Depression and Costs of Health Care." *Psychosomatics* 50 (4): 392–401.

Wells, K. B., C. Sherbourne, M. Schoenbaum, N. Duan, L. Meredith, J. Unutzer . . . L. V. Rubenstein. 2000. "Impact of Disseminating Quality Improvement Programs for Depression in Managed Primary Care: A Randomized Controlled Trial." *JAMA* 283 (2): 212–20.

Weng, H. Y., A. S. Fox, A. J. Shackman, D. E. Stodola, J.Z.K. Caldwell, M. C. Olson, . . . R. J. Davidson. 2013. "Compassion Training Alters Altruism and Neural Responses to Suffering." *Psychological Science* 24 (7): 1171–80.

Wessely, S. 2007. "A Defence of the Randomized Controlled Trial in Mental Health." *Biosocieties* 2 (1): 115–27.

West, P., and H. Sweeting. 2003. "Fifteen, Female, and Stressed: Changing Patterns of Psychological Distress over Time." *Journal of Child Psychology and Psychiatry* 44 (3): 399–411.

Whooley, M. A., P. de Jonge, E. Vittinghoff, C. Otte, R. Moos, R. M. Carney, . . . W. S. Browner. 2008. "Depressive Symptoms, Health Behaviors, and Risk of Cardiovascular Events in Patients with Coronary Heart Disease." *JAMA* 300 (20): 2379–88.

Wilkinson, R., and K. Pickett. 2009. *The Spirit Level: Why More Equal Societies Almost Always Do Better*. London: Allen Lane.

Williams, J.M.G. 2001. *Suicide and Attempted Suicide*. London: Penguin.

Williams, J.M.G., and J. Kabat-Zinn, eds. 2013. *Mindfulness: Diverse Perspectives on Its Meaning, Origins, and Applications*. London: Routledge.

Williams, J.M.G., and D. Penman. 2011. *Mindfulness: A Practical Guide to Finding Peace in a Frantic World*. London: Piatkus.

Wilson, B. 2008. *Decency and Disorder: The Age of Cant, 1789–1837*. London: Faber.

Wilson, G. T., and C. G Fairburn. 2007. "Treatments for Eating Disorders." In *A Guide to Treatments That Work*, 3rd ed., edited by P. E. Nathan, and J. M. Gorman. New York: Oxford University Press.

Wilson, S., T. Benton, E. Scott, and L. Kendall. 2007. *London Challenge: Survey of Pupils and Teachers 2006*. Slough: National Foundation for Educational Research.

Wilson, T. D. 2011. *Redirect: The Surprising New Science of Psychological Change*. London: Allen Lane.

Wittchen, H.-U., M. Fuetsch, H. Sonntag, N. Muller, and M. Liebowitz. 1999. "Disability and Quality of Life in Pure and Comorbid Social Phobia: Findings from a Controlled Study." *European Psychiatry* 14 (3): 118–31.

Wittchen, H.-U., and F. Jacobi. 2005. "Size and Burden of Mental Disorders in Europe: A Critical Review and Appraisal of 27 Studies." *European Neuropsychopharmacology* 15: 357–76.

Wolpe, J. 1958. *Psychotherapy through Reciprocal Inhibition*. Palo Alto, CA: Stanford University Press.

Wolpert, L. 1999. *Malignant Sadness: The Anatomy of Depression*. New York: Free Press.

Wolpert, M., P. Fuggle, D. Cottrell, P. Fonagy, J. Phillips, S. Pilling, . . . M. Target. 2006. *Drawing on the Evidence: Advice for Mental Health Professionals Working with Children and Adolescents*. 2nd ed. CAMHS Publications.

Worell, J., ed. 2002. *Encyclopedia of Women and Gender: Sex Similarities and Differences and the Impact of Society on Gender*, vol. 1. San Diego: Academic Press.

World Economic Forum (WEF). 2012. *Well-Being and Global Success: A Report Prepared by the World Economic Forum Global Agenda Council on Health and Well-Being*. Geneva.

World Health Organization (WHO). 2002. *World Report on Violence and Health*, edited by E. G. Krug, L. L. Dahlberg, J. A. Mercy, A. B. Zwi, and R. Lozano. Geneva.

———. 2003. *Caring for Children and Adolescents with Mental Disorders: Setting WHO Directions*. Geneva.

———. 2004. *Prevention of Mental Disorders: Effective Interventions and Policy Options*. Geneva.

———. 2008. *The Global Burden of Disease: 2004 Update*. Geneva.

Wulsin, L. R., J. C. Evans, R. S. Vasan, J. M. Murabito, M. Kelly-Hayes, and E. J. Benjamin. 2005. "Depressive Symptoms, Coronary Heart Disease, and Overall Mortality in the Framingham Heart Study." *Psychosomatic Medicine* 67: 697–702.

Young Minds. 2011. "Cuts Begin to Bite for Some." *Young Minds Magazine* 113: 25–27.

INDEX

Page numbers in italics refer to pages with charts or tables on them. The names of national leaders may refer to the individual or the administration or both.

31901056620570